NEW RITUALS FOR OLD

New Rituals for Old

Nursing through the Looking Glass

Pauline Ford RGN, DHSM, CMS
*Royal College of Nursing Adviser in Nursing and Older People,
Royal College of Nursing, London*

and

Mike Walsh BA, PGCE, RGN, DipN
*Head of the Department of Nursing and Midwifery Studies,
St. Martin's College, Lancaster*

Foreword by Christine Hancock BSc(Econ), RGN
General Secretary, Royal College of Nursing, London

Cartoons by Kipper Williams

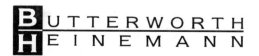

Butterworth-Heinemann Ltd
Linacre House, Jordan Hill, Oxford OX2 8DP

℞ A member of the Reed Elsevier plc group

OXFORD   LONDON   BOSTON
NEW DELHI   SINGAPORE   SYDNEY
TOKYO   TORONTO   WELLINGTON

First published 1994
Reprinted 1995 (twice)

British Library Cataloguing in Publication Data
Ford, Pauline
New Rituals for Old: Nursing through the
looking glass
I. Title   II. Walsh, Mike
610.73

ISBN 0 7506 1581 8

Library of Congress Cataloging in Publication Data
Ford, Pauline.
New rituals for old: nursing though the looking glass/Pauline
Ford and Mike Walsh: foreword by Christine Hancock.
p.   cm.
Includes bibliographical references and index.
ISBN 0 7506 1581 8
1. Nursing – Practice.   2. Nursing – Philosophy.   3. Nurses – Job
satisfaction.   I. Walsh, Mike.   II. Title.
RT82.F555
610.73–dc20   93–46155
                                          CIP

Typeset by TecSet Ltd, Wallington, Surrey
Printed and bound in Great Britain by
Biddles Ltd, Guildford and King's Lynn

Contents

Foreword by Christine Hancock   vii
Preface   ix

Part One   Concepts of Empowerment   1

 1 Of prophets and false messiahs: which way to
    the promised land?   3
 2 Empowering the nurse: a feminist perspective   25
 3 Empowerment, nursing and clinical practice   41
 4 Nursing and change   58
 5 Liberation nursing   84

Part Two   The Delivery of Care   93

 6 Questions of quality   95
 7 Primary nursing   125
 8 The nurse practitioner   155
 9 Care plans, process and models   181
10 The nursing process: time for a change?   210
11 A case study of nursing empowerment   228
12 Reflections   241

Index   251

Foreword

In 1989, with *Nursing Rituals: Research and Rational Actions*, Pauline Ford and Mike Walsh challenged us all to shake off the comfortable complacency of routine and ritual and to take a fresh look at nursing practice.

They demonstrated, in a frank, thought provoking but very readable book, just how much routine nursing practice was being conducted not on the basis of sound research but because it had 'always been done that way'.

Five years on, they are asking us to pause and reflect on whether we are in danger of substituting new rituals for old. Nursing has been subjected to a battery of changes over the last decade, some managerial, some political, some practice led.

Most of those changes have been imposed on, rather than owned by nurses themselves. Pauline and Mike argue that because nursing is not in control of its own destiny, nurses tend to ritualize new approaches to care so that the care plan or the nursing process become empty procedures, as redundant as the old bath book.

Pauline and Mike warn against false messiahs. Perhaps they need to remember the old adage that prophets are never recognized in their own country.

Nursing is not good at accommodating dissent and those who question old or new orthodoxies make uncomfortable colleagues. They have dared to open up some relatively new but well-established ideas and practices to critical scrutiny.

Primary nursing, quality assurance, the development of nurse practitioners, care plans and nursing models are all subjected to clear sighted examination and analysis. In the process a great deal of muddled thinking and ritualistic behaviour is uncovered.

Just what do we mean by primary nursing?, they ask. Is it a particular method of organizing nursing care, a patient centred philosophy of care or an amorphous bundle of aspirations for good practice?

Is the nursing process and the writing of care plans a constraint upon the experienced and expert nurse of little tangible benefit to the patient?

But the authors are emphatically not 'getting at' nurses. They offer a powerful critique of nursing's traditional occupational power-lessness. They use feminist insights and the perspective of social theorist Paulo Freire to show how oppressed groups participate in their own subordination.

And they offer a vision of empowerment, liberation nursing, which builds on the work of Freire, Schon and Benner.

They show how nursing can learn to value its own knowledge base, how nurses can empower themselves and effect lasting change. Through empowerment, concepts of real value, like the RCN's own approach to standard setting, like primary nursing and nurse practitioners, can become a liberating force within nursing, not a new constraint.

It is a source of great pleasure to see these two authors collaborating again on a new attempt to shake up the world of nursing. Pauline and Mike met through a very powerful empower-ing network – the Royal College of Nursing – which offers nurses a unique forum for discussion, support, personal and professional growth and a platform to work for the empowerment of nursing.

I commend this book to all nurses who want to understand the complex nature of nursing and to change it for the better.

Christine Hancock
General Secretary,
Royal College of Nursing

Preface

Nursing practice was critiqued in our first book, *Nursing Rituals: Research and Rational Actions* (Butterworth-Heinemann, 1989) for persisting with unthinking ritual rather than validated, research-based actions. Many new concepts have however been introduced into nursing in the last decade or so. The concern of these two authors is that many of these brave new ideas have been embraced in an uncritical manner and consequently are in danger of becoming as ritualized as salt in the bathwater or the bedpan round.

In this book we have held up concepts such as primary nursing and quality assurance to the harsh glare of critical enquiry. Research findings have been analysed and utilized in this critical process. The results challenge conventional wisdom about some recent nursing developments and set out a series of arguments which have to be answered. It is only in this way, by engaging the proponents of new nursing ideas in critical debate, that nursing can avoid repeating the mistakes of the past and ritualizing many potentially powerful and beneficial ideas.

We have also set out to synthesize ideas from differing areas in a way that can liberate and empower clinical nursing. The work of Donald Schon in the field of the reflective practitioner links to Pat Benner's work on expert nursing. When these powerful ideas are synthesized with the emancipating insights that are derived from the writings of critical social theorists such as Paulo Freire and also various feminist writers, the result is a new approach to nursing that we have dubbed 'liberation nursing'.

The book therefore poses a double challenge to the reader. We critically question perceived wisdom concerning new ideas and also dare the reader to go further in pursuit of empowerment and liberation for nursing. The new millenium beckons and we are hoping that clinical nurses are ready to throw off the oppression of tradition and authority once and for all in pursuit of professional autonomy.

Pauline Ford
Mike Walsh

PART ONE

Concepts of
Empowerment

1 Of prophets and false messiahs: which way to the promised land?

Shabbatai Zevi is a little-known but fascinating historical figure. He lived in the mid 17th century in what is now Turkey and he convinced large numbers of Jewish people that he was indeed the messiah come to lead them to the promised land. He was the latest in a long line of such messiahs who appeared in central and eastern Europe during historical times, convincing an oppressed and persecuted people, the Jews, that he was the messiah and had all the answers that would make life better.

His predecessors had been avidly believed, in direct proportion to the plight and gullibility of their audiences and also to the degree of oppression they were suffering. Each messiah in turn had proved false and Shabbatai Zevi, perhaps the most charismatic of these men, was to leave his followers even more aggrieved than the others as he converted to Islam and renounced all his previous claims to be the messiah the Jewish people had been waiting for down the ages. The Turkish authorities 'persuaded' him that they could not allow such dissension within the empire and, given a choice between death and conversion to Islam, he chose Islam.

Whole villages and communities had been taken in by his claims. Poor families had all their worldly possessions packed and were awaiting the word to follow their messiah to the promised land, a word that never came. Instead, three centuries later, as we know, the Jewish people are making their own promised land the hard way in the modern state of Israel, without any messianic leaders.

The reader may now be wondering if this book has accidently found its way into the wrong section of the bookshop and has been picked up by mistake. The answer is no, and we hope that a moment's reflection might allow you to see that this tale is relevant to nursing today. The main theme of this book is that nurses should not meekly follow 'experts' but instead value themselves and the wisdom of their patients. Critical self-examination and reflection upon practice provide the means for nursing's future development, not following charismatic 'messiahs' who appear to have all the answers.

Nurses have traditionally been oppressed by virtue of being predominantly women in a patriarchal society and also by virtue of being seen as handmaidens to the powerful medical profession. Nursing lacks a history of scholarly and academic development to rank alongside other disciplines such as medicine, law or the natural sciences. The lack of an in-depth theoretical framework leaves nursing vulnerable not only to ritualistic practice but also, paradoxically, to unsubstantiated 'big new ideas' preached with messianic zeal in certain quarters. Within the last decade or two, ideas such as primary nursing and nursing models have exploded on to the normally conservative health care and nursing scene. They have been seized on as the answer to all our problems by many but some of the proponents of such ideas may, like Shabbatai Zevi, turn out to be false prophets as their untried ideas have been accepted without question.

The patron saint of nursing might well be St Paul, given the number of conversions on the road to Damascus that have dramatically taken place as nurses, educationalists and managers have suddenly embraced a range of new ideas with far more conviction than the supporting evidence would suggest was wise. As we shall demonstrate in subsequent chapters, however good the ideas might be, the evidence to support changing to primary nursing, the nursing process or nursing models does not exist. Charismatic individuals and high-powered marketing strategies

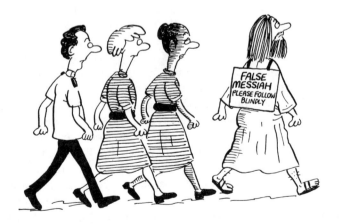

have appeared in association with these bright new ideas, in such a way that they may appear to be the new messiahs of health care. The question therefore raises itself: are these messiahs distant cousins of Shabbatai Zevi? Should not nursing and the way we organize health care be developing its theoretical base in a more rational way, rather than looking for messiahs?

The authors have argued already that some nursing care is of little value and some may actually be harmful due to the unthinking ritualistic way in which it is carried out and the lack of any rational basis for many nursing actions (Walsh and Ford, 1989). The danger is that many new and potentially valuable innovations could go down the road to ritualization if they are accepted without question. Nursing developments could become devalued and debased by unthinking acceptance. A dependence upon messianic and charismatic leadership is as dangerous as burying our collective heads in the sand and hoping the need to change will just go away.

Nursing needs a way of approaching change, a way of thinking about and conceptualizing nursing, a way of moving forwards away from tradition and ritual, but developing in a rational way in which nurses can justify their actions and only implement change when it is subject to evaluation and scrutiny to check it has had a beneficial effect. This need for a framework on which we can construct the discipline of nursing and build systems that encourage innovative practice (which has a reasonable chance of producing better care) has been likened elsewhere (Walsh, 1991) to a map laying out the territory of nursing. Without such a set of charts and maps we are left with unthinking ritual on the one hand and naïve acceptance of bright new ideas on the other – new rituals for old, as we suggest in the title.

Our main argument is that the blind acceptance of grand new ideas will benefit patients as little as traditional care, for they may in themselves eventually become ritualistic and spawn a whole new generation of rituals. Innovation is crucial to the future of nursing, but only when new ideas are worked through in a thoughtful, questioning way rather than blindly accepted with the fervour and unquestioning faith normally accorded to profound religious revelations.

This book will endeavour to explore areas where we feel this is happening today. We seek to ask awkward questions and in the process make nurses think about what they are doing and why they

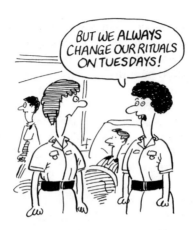

are so readily accepting one idea but rejecting another. Ideas are powerful things, as Victor Hugo recognized in his *Histoire d'un Crime (La Chute)* when he wrote that:

A stand can be made against invasion by an army; no stand can be made against the invasion by an idea.

It is the invasion of nursing by some ideas which seem to sweep all before them, despite lacking any supporting evidence, that we are critical of. So we will ask awkward questions and challenge big new ideas. It would be as wrong to close the frontiers to new ideas as it would be to welcome every new idea with open arms and enthusiastically rush into its embrace. Echoing Victor Hugo, we are arguing for a few border controls and passport checks to satisfy ourselves of the merits of bright new ideas before allowing them free access to the body of nursing!

Rituals today and their origins

In order to explore the whole area of ritualistic health care in this way, the point of departure needs to be a brief account of what is meant by ritualistic care and how it originated in nursing.

In our first book on this subject (Walsh and Ford, 1989) we argued that much clinical nursing lacked a rational basis and frequently ignored research findings which were at times completely contrary to practice. The first question this raises is, of course, why? Why should educated, hard-working and highly motivated, respected, caring professionals behave in such an unprofessional way, which may be positively harmful at times to their clients? The following possible reasons, acting together in varying degrees, may offer some explanation of this nursing paradox:

- Training rather than education.
- Gender stereotyping.
- The immature state of research and research awareness.
- Stress defence mechanisms.
- The influence of attitudes and beliefs.

Education and training
There is a fundamental difference between training and education and, until recently, nurses received the former, not the latter. Put simply, a dog is *trained* to perform tricks but a biology graduate is *educated* in the science of biology.

Training is characterized by the ability to perform tasks correctly and efficiently; it is about obedience, the prompt carrying-out of orders and it can be performed cheaply for large numbers of trainees in the workplace. Training may be appropriate for animals without the brain power of humans; it may be appropriate for getting humans to perform tasks involving inanimate objects that do not interact with the human operator (e.g. bricks and mortar), but is training appropriate for working with other humans who are all individuals, who ask questions, have rights and their own point of view? Working with human beings in a therapeutic relationship involves thinking, the asking and answering of questions such as why?

Training does not usually address the issue of why? It may not even properly address the issue of how? Training typically gives one way of doing a task without equipping the trainee with the necessary critical faculties to look at alternatives or the under-standing to adapt a particular solution to a different situation. Questions may be seen as getting in the way of training because they require answers, high-level cognitive skills and a knowledge base that extends beyond the procedure manual. Questions cannot be credibly answered in a professional context by saying 'Because I said so' or 'We always do it that way'.

Training tends to produce single, standard answers to problems; routine solutions lead to routine actions – rituals. There is a premium on the technical skills of a task rather than asking the question: does this task need to be done at all? Some nurses pride themselves on their dressing techniques, following the procedure manual to the letter, but do they ask whether the techniques used are appropriate, necessary or beneficial to the patient?

Education, on the other hand, is about developing a flexible enquiring mind able to approach a situation from different angles. The individual should be able to consider alternative solutions within a critical and analytical framework, utilizing a strong knowledge base, before deciding on a solution to a problem or a course of action. This is recognized by Benner (1984) as a key stage in the development of an expert nurse, though she argues that to be an expert, the nurse needs to progress beyond this analytical stage. Benner's work will be discussed further in Chapter 3.

Education therefore equips the nurse to consider alternatives and decide a course of action unique to each situation. Creativity and flexibility should be the hallmarks of education in action. However, if the nurse has been trained to be an efficient performer of tasks, trained to follow the narrow confines of the procedure manual, trained to see only the standard solution to a problem and questions and alternative suggestions are frowned on, then unthinking and ritualistic care is the likely outcome.

It is not too difficult to see how this love affair with procedures, routines and training originated in nursing. Modern nursing history starts in Victorian times with Miss Nightingale in the Crimean war. The military environment in which early nursing began would have been characterized by the notion that orders were to be given and obeyed. Miss Nightingale returned from the wars to a Victorian Britain that was an extremely patriarchal society: women were expected to obey the head of the household at all times. These two factors alone probably ensured that obedience was a key characteristic of the early nurse, and obedience is a much more comfortable bedfellow with training than education.

Nursing in the 20th century followed the apprenticeship model of training. This meant that hospitals could be run at low cost using large numbers of apprentice nurses as cheap labour. One consequence of depending so heavily upon students was that the work-force became increasingly transient; a large part of the ward team were never on the ward for more than a month or two as the students rotated their way through the different wards, often in a chaotic way that had little resemblance to whatever theory they were being taught during blocks in the school.

Students therefore had little chance to relate theory to practice and, from the ward sister's point of view, the priority was getting the work done. The efficient way of meeting this goal with a rapidly changing work force was training in standard solutions, procedures and tasks, with little or no time to explain why it was done this way or how something might be done differently. Task-focused training got the work done when a large part of the workforce was transient.

Linking these themes together, it is not difficult to see how the training model evolved within nursing rather than an educational approach to learning.

A similar pattern is discerned by American authors. Meleis (1991) has written of student nurses being used as cheap labour within an apprenticeship system, leading to nursing being subordinated to tasks with little time for thought or reflection. The logical consequence of this system, as Meleis observes, was that nurses adopted subservient attitudes and an unquestioning acceptance of authority. Chinn and Jacobs (1987) consider that for most of the 20th century nursing practice was based upon rules and traditions operating within an apprenticeship system. They comment upon the lack of testing of such rules and procedures and their unquestioning acceptance. The apprentice nurse merely observes what goes on and copies the way things are done whilst at the same time memorizing the rules for procedures. It is not surprising therefore that there was a lack of what might be called a body of nursing knowledge comparable to any other discipline and that from this background unthinking and ritualistic care developed.

The situation was further exacerbated by the employment of large numbers of nursing assistants who often had relatively low levels of educational achievement at school and who had no formal teaching in nursing at all. The focus was very much upon on-the-job training in how to do tasks and, as the nursing assistant tended to stay on the same ward, it was from her that students often learnt during their period on any one ward. Most nursing assistants are well-motivated and caring people, but they lack any formal nursing education and have a narrow perspective on care, stemming from limited experience. Dependence upon assistants limits the delivery of care to very narrow, standardized pathways. York Centre for Health Economics (1992) showed that high standards of care depend upon using a high proportion of qualified staff. This need not cost more, as fewer staff overall need to be employed, contradicting the views of some managers who naïvely think they can save money by employing a large number of unqualified staff. Dependence upon staff who are lacking education not only leads to ritualistic care but also is not cost-effective.

The influence of gender stereotyping

In the previous section, the dominance of training rather than education in the field of nursing was seen as contributing towards ritualistic practice. The evolution of modern nursing as predominantly women's work in a male-dominated society has also made a major contribution towards unthinking obedience to orders and hence ritualistic practice.

Female nurses were subordinated to male dominance both by virtue of being female in a patriarchal society and also by being seen as assistants to the male-dominated medical profession. The stereotype of the loyal subordinate, following orders and complying with instructions is not consistent with an autonomous professional, yet that is how nursing has largely been through the 20th century. Nurses did as they were told by doctors, just as wives were expected until recently to love, honour and *obey* their husbands! With this extent of socialization into subordinate roles, it is not surprising that following orders and procedures became the norm, and so ritualistic practice came to be the dominant mode of care, rather than questioning, innovative and autonomous professionalism.

There is some interesting transatlantic support for this stereotypical view of nursing from the work of Kaler *et al.* (1989), who interviewed a sample of 110 adults in a shopping mall in California. They asked subjects to rate various professions in terms of educational levels and other characteristics. The researchers were able to develop a scale running from high-achievement orientation to a strong-helping orientation which also corresponded to an axis measuring male–female characteristics (Figure 1.1). Nursing was perceived by the public as lying far towards the helping/female end of the scale, while at the same time requiring a lower level of education than the average repair person. When compared to doctors, nurses were seen as less logical, intelligent or extrovert and less able to show leadership. The authors conclude that the public sees nurses in terms which are consensually acknowledged as typically feminine and also that nursing needs to assert the right to practise so that there can be another stereotype of nursing in the public's mind – intelligent and autonomous.

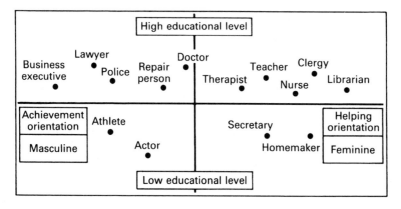

Figure 1.1 *Two-dimensional solution for similarities of 14 occupations (Levy et al., 1989, reproduced with permission)*

This work is of course American and cannot therefore be readily transposed into the UK without entering the caveat that the British public might see nurses differently. However, from the evidence in the media, it is likely that UK perceptions would not be too different from those reported in this study.

Nurse authors have recently begun to discuss the effects of gender upon nursing's attempts to develop as a profession in its own right. Lumby (1991) rightly points out the major problem of the word 'nurse' and its derivation from the Greek word meaning to nurture or nourish which, when seen as suckling the young, is an essentially female activity. She observes that other professions do not have the disadvantage of this gender label stuck to their titles (e.g. doctor, teacher, etc.). Nursing was therefore seen as women's work *par excellence* and Lumby suggests that the increasing numbers of men entering nursing in the last couple of decades is a contributory factor towards its belated professionalization.

A central tenet of feminism is that women are an oppressed group and consequently it is logical to see nurses, being predominantly female, as also being oppressed (Speedy, 1991). Oppressed groups do not have the opportunity to develop their own consciousness, their own ethos, but rather have the ways of the oppressor imposed upon them. It might subvert the system and deprive those in power of the thing they most desire – power! The analogies with nursing are obvious as the male-dominated medical profession for so long controlled the training of nurses, thereby ensuring they learnt only what doctors felt it fitting for their assistants to know. The last couple of decades have seen nursing break free from its medical shackles, only to be ensnared by another powerful male-dominated group – managers.

Nursing lost its managerial control of nursing with the introduction of general management in the mid 1980s and government restructuring has since increased the power of – predominantly male – business managers and accountants over nurses. If medical domination was thought of as a benign dictatorship, the macho management styles being encountered today have a much more malign feel to them.

The result is the same – nurses, a predominantly female group, are being told what they can and cannot do by men who are not nurses, and at times being made redundant by them. Oppression is a good word to describe such activity, and the oppressed are never free to try out new ideas or receive an education that stimulates questions and dissent. Survival as an oppressed person requires conformity, an ability to follow orders and not ask questions – all of which lead to unthinking and ritualistic practice. Blow the whistle and be assertive at your peril!

If nurses are to move away from ritualistic care, increased self-awareness and assertiveness is essential, as well as a concerted attack upon nursing stereotypes. Slater (1990) has described how nurses were traditionally trained to be acquiescent and submissive, the opposites of what an education would have produced. To be assertive, Slater continues, the nurse needs to define herself and, if the only definition we have of nursing is in the traditional female, subservient role, then nurses will not make much progress down the road to assertiveness.

The male-dominated society in which we live frowns upon assertive women. As if this is not enough of a handicap for nursing, there is evidence that whatever assertiveness women may have is socialized out of them in the nursing workplace. Gerry (1989) has reported upon a study which found that nurses gave less assertive responses to questionnaires constructed around workplace scenarios compared to everyday life. This research has the limitation of being based upon interviews and questionnaires, i.e. what the subjects said they would do if a situation occurred, rather than observation of what they actually did, but has the strength of being based upon a substantial sample of 99 nurses.

It is worrying that the lower levels of assertiveness associated with being female are further reduced when in the work situation. Gerry found that there was a clear rank order of assertiveness scores from Sisters down to Enrolled Nurses, who came last. She also reported that knowledge, confidence, experience and the wearing of uniform promoted assertiveness, whilst tradition, training and the hierarchical structure were reported as the main inhibitors of assertiveness. Seen in this light, perhaps the wearing of uniform promotes assertiveness by reducing the assertiveness of the subordinate party? The hospital system, due to the clear position established in the hierarchy by the different uniforms, seems to work to reduce assertive behaviour in female nurses overall when compared to everyday life – a key finding of Gerry's research.

Graham (1984) has pointed out that in a male-dominated society females learn to care for others rather than themselves, at the expense of their own self-image. Does this matter? Ask any nurse who has tried to introduce a change, and been confronted by the steamroller of managerial authority and the answer is that it does matter. Nursing will never be able to change its practice if nurses do not value themselves sufficiently and have the necessary assertiveness to persuade, cajole or use a whole host of other change strategems to implement innovation at the expense of tradition and ritual. It also matters if we care about the rights and wrongs of oppression and exploitation.

Slater (1990) has described some interesting work in assertiveness training done with groups of nurses in which inequalities within the NHS between men and women, doctors and nurses became apparent. Self-esteem and assertive behaviour were found to be closely interdependent. Differences in assumed rights related to gender were clear: females often played a sort of game to let males get their own way in order to protect the male ego. This of course negates the self-worth of females and, by extrapolation, nursing as a whole.

In summarizing the benefits of the assertiveness training workshops that she runs, Slater has argued that they promote openness, trust, constructive feedback and a high degree of flexibility, which in turn allow people to assert themselves. The development of nursing practice away from slavish obedience to the procedure manual surely depends upon the sort of characteristics that Slater suggests are associated with assertiveness. Openness and flexibility allow the nurse to think of new ideas while trust permits other staff to feel able to try them out and constructive feedback is crucial to evaluating their effectiveness.

The gender stereotypes that go with being female have held nursing back in its attempts to develop as a profession and have inhibited the growth of scholarly activity amongst nurses. The world view of many men – that women should do as they are told and not ask questions – prevents the growth of an enquiring professional mind and leads instead to reliance upon tradition and ritual. This becomes a self-fulfilling prophecy as men can say that nurses are unable to show the sort of characteristics that allow them to be taken seriously as professionals and academics within the field of nursing. They are easily dismissed as of little importance. The real trick in this sytem is that as it is men who define the characteristics of academia, the objective rationalism of science, the ground rules for success are literally man-made. The feminist movement has an alternative view of research and scholarly activity, which will be discussed in Chapter 2.

Research

Research is a key that opens the door to the development of any profession. In nursing, however, this key seems to have initially been tried in the wrong door and latterly, even though the correct door has been located, it appears to have encountered a very rusty lock. If nursing is to progress away from ritualistic practice, the role of research therefore deserves considerable attention.

Nursing was originally hampered by a lack of research, for, as we shall see later, the absence of research severely limits the development of key areas of knowledge. Practice was based on tradition with little or no systematic evaluation of the effectiveness of care given. This was an authoritarian type of knowing: the nurse knew what to do because s/he was told what to do by a senior figure in the hierarchy.

In the 1950s and 1960s, research first began to look at nursing, but not at clinical nursing for, as Meleis (1991) points out, the key issues were administrative in nature, such as workforce planning, wastage rates and training programmes. The key was being tried in the wrong door as far as reforming clinical practice was concerned. Those responsible for the delivery of health care had woken up to the enormous costs of nurse training and salaries to the health budget. It must be added that this was due more to the large numbers of nurses involved, as nursing was, and is, very labour-intensive. This large cost was not born of high salaries for each individual nurse! Research investigated the large-scale picture and even began to look at why nurses left nursing, but the very stuff of nursing, clinical practice, remained hidden away from the enquiring eye, behind the screens of tradition and mythology.

Few nurses were equipped with the necessary skills of research or were even aware that it existed. Consequently researchers with a clinical base simply did not exist. Research remained something that only doctors did and nurses need not bother themselves with, even if they had the time, which they usually did not, such were the rigorous demands of ward routine.

The 1970s saw change in the air. The first degree courses in nursing were at last beginning to produce nurses who had been educated rather than trained. They had been introduced to research as a means of discovery and validating practice; they had been taught to query and ask why. The Royal College of Nursing led the way with a major series of research projects which have become classics in their own time, such as Smith's work on preoperative fasting (1972) and Hayward's work on postoperative pain (1975).

At last nurses were investigating clinical nursing. This work has been followed by significant efforts aimed at researching clinical nursing over the last decade or so, yet ritualistic care continues to bedevil practice. Why, 15 years after all this pioneering research, could the present authors (Walsh and Ford, 1989) find so much evidence of this classic early work being ignored? The research key is now in the right lock, but it has failed to open the door to progressive practice. The following suggestions might explain why the lock is proving so obstinate.

For any new way of thinking to have an impact, its value has to be accepted by those at whom it is directed. A study of research methods and the value of research was the exception rather than the rule in nurse training during the 1970s and on into the 1980s. Typical of these welcome exceptions were post basic part-time courses such as the University of London Diploma in Nursing (1983 syllabus) and CNAA-validated Diplomas in Professional Studies which began to introduce in-depth studies in research methodology to small numbers of nurses during the 1980s, while English Nursing Board courses also made nurses aware of the potential of research. These programmes affected only a small proportion of nurses, and it has taken the development of nursing education with the Project 2000 initiative and the spread of degree courses in the last few years to start to produce a whole new generation of nurses for whom research is a natural part of nursing from the very beginning of their education.

The net result of nursing's reluctance to incorporate research into the learning process of its practitioners has been to propagate ritualistic and unthinking practice. Nurses have been unable to investigate the effectiveness of care and look for new methods of care delivery because they did not have the essential tools needed for such intellectual activity – the tools of the researcher.

Worse still, now that research into clinical nursing is finally taking place, many nurses seem unable or unwilling to base their practice upon that research. History has left us with a significant number of nurses who do not have the academic skills to appreciate the significance of research findings or who are unaware that the findings exist at all because they do not read research papers. The situation is compounded by some researchers who write up their work in pseudoscientific jargon that forms a forbidding and impenetrable barrier to understanding. There is no point in research if the findings are inaccessible to the people who most need to know what those findings are. This is no place for academic snobbery, but rather for plain English.

The absence of clinical research from nursing's agenda has contributed therefore to much ritualistic practice and even today, when research is being carried out, there are whole generations of nurses to whom research is something of an unknown quantity. A major effort to raise nursing's awareness of research must accompany any research initiatives in order that the results of academic enquiry may be translated into clinical practice.

Stress defence mechanisms

Few people would dispute the assertion that nursing is a stressful occupation. Chapman (1983) has suggested that the origins of much ritualistic practice lies in nurses finding ways to cope with these stresses. Chapman carried out a largely covert observational piece of research in a range of London hospitals, observing ritualistic practice at first hand, and was able to link what she saw to stress defence mechanisms amongst the nurses that she worked with.

Support for this view may be found within the field of psychology. Pitts and Phillips (1991), for example, in reviewing the literature on mechanisms used for coping with stress, discuss avoidance strategies where the person copes with stressful stimuli by avoiding them. The nurse thus avoids the stresses of being close to a patient by carrying out a series of often unnecessary tasks that allow avoidance or, if in close contact while, for example, attending to personal hygiene, does so in a busy mechanistic way that inhibits meaningful conversation.

Another way of looking at stress coping strategies is to see them as either problem-focused or emotion-focused (Atkinson *et al.*, 1987). In the former the person tries to deal rationally with the problem causing the stress and in the latter the person concentrates on dealing with the emotions generated by the stress while ignoring the cause or problem. This view readily translates to the clinical situation where stress is present all the time as patients may suffer pain, disfigurement or death. Rather than deal with the source of the stress which is the patient's condition (problem-focused coping), nurses may tend to deal with the emotions produced in themselves and find strategies to deaden those feelings (emotion-focused coping). Successful strategies are to be very busy, avoid meaningful conversations and follow procedures mechanistically without having to think about what is being done and why. In this way nurses dull the emotions produced by stressful situations; rituals act as an anaesthetic to deaden the pain caused by real patient problems.

This view of stress coping behaviour presents a major challenge to initiatives such as care planning and primary nursing which, to be successful, require the nurse to be close to the patient, working with the individual to deal with a whole range of stressful problems. Are we asking too much of the nurse to expect him or her to take on board the problems of a group of patients in this way? Doctors can deal with these sort of difficulties by using distance as a defence because they may only see the patient for a few minutes each day. Further, the biomedical model ensures that the doctor's attention is focused upon only a malfunctioning biological component within an interconnected series of systems, not a whole person. Once we start to look holistically at a person and get very close to that person for 8 hours a day and carry responsibility for what happens to them for the other 16 hours as their primary nurse, the stresses become very great indeed.

If ritualistic behaviour evolved as a means of coping with the stresses of nursing and if changes such as primary nursing are likely to increase those stresses, the future looks set to see an increase in ritualistic practice. Nursing needs therefore to recognize the stresses that are involved in itself and develop more effective coping mechanisms in its practitioners. Nurses need to be free to admit that they find things difficult or else we add the burden of guilt to the stresses with which the individual is struggling to cope. Stress management needs to become an essential part of nursing education and, crucially, of nursing practice, if initiatives such as primary nursing are to succeed and if ritualistic, unthinking care is to become a thing of the past.

A final thought might be directed at managers who aim for impressive throughput statistics: they should pause to consider the hidden costs of overburdened nursing staff and the impact this has on standards of care. Workload clearly affects stress levels and managers need to address this question of stress with a more constructive approach if they are to get the best out of their workforce in the long run.

There is also a thought here for clinical nurses: do you need to be doing everything that you are doing? Might not the reason why nurses feel overworked be that some of what they do is not necessary – it is a ritual, a tradition, but not necessary. As Walsh and Ford have argued (1989), time spent stripping every bed on the ward every morning might be better spent doing other things, with the result that current staffing levels may not be as inadequate as they might appear.

Attitudes and beliefs in nursing

There is one remaining area that is worthy of exploration if possible causes for ritualistic nursing practice are to be discovered and this can best be approached via the question: how do we know what we know? If a body of knowledge is built up by research and enquiry, testing and evaluating ideas, then it is open to challenge and change. However, if a body of knowledge is really little more than beliefs, opinions and attitudes handed down in a hierarchical way, then challenge and change will tend to be stifled as the dead hand of tradition and obedience guides practice along ritualistic tramlines. Nursing carries around a significant amount of baggage that falls into this latter category, hence the problem of ritualistic practice.

Much of the conventional wisdom passed on in nurse training has been little more than personal beliefs, prejudices and attitudes, rather than something that would be recognized as knowledge in any other discipline. In that sense, nursing has had more in common with religion than an academic activity.

Attitudes are likes and dislikes about things. They are associated with beliefs about the object in question and behaviours which flow from the attitude (Atkinson *et al.*, 1987). There is therefore a three-component system – affective (attitude), cognitive (belief) and behavioural (action). For example, task-oriented care may be observed on a ward as a behaviour that is associated with the belief that it 'gets the work done', which links with the attitude that getting a list of tasks performed is a good thing. This method of organizing nursing care, however, is not founded in any rational knowledge base or derived from any way of knowing which is the best way of delivering care – it is a product of beliefs and attitudes.

In answering the question of why people have attitudes, Hewstone *et al.* (1988) suggest that it might be more profitable to explore a slightly different question: what are the results of holding attitudes? In the view of these authors, four main explanations can be found in the literature, the first of which is a Freudian explanation couched in terms of attitudes being an ego defence mechanism. They may also be seen as permitting us to express our own core values and therefore reinforce our self-concept. Attitudes might also allow us to be liked by others for if we express similar attitudes to others, it is more probable that they will like us. Finally, attitudes allow us to make sense of a complicated world by categorizing incoming information into familiar mental pigeonholes.

These explanations of why people hold attitudes strike resonant chords within nursing. Nurses who qualified some years ago may feel threatened by students and bright, newly qualified staff, therefore holding on to and developing strong attitudes helps to defend the nurse's sense of ego. Nurses tend to feel strongly about their work and therefore the need to express core values in often difficult situations is essential, coupled with the need to hang on to a self-concept which is often severely battered by the real world of the NHS in the 1990s. Attitudes are therefore an important way of reinforcing a nurse's values and surviving in stressful circumstances. The third view of attitude formation is consistent with the process of socialization in nursing: adopting the prevailing attitudes of those in authority makes it easier for the student and junior staff nurse to survive. Finally, there are few who would disagree that life for the nurse can be very hectic, with a great deal of new information having to be absorbed and made sense of every day. Attitudes therefore help the nurse make sense of a complex working environment.

From the above analysis, it seems that each of these four explanations of the development of attitudes and beliefs fits the mainstream of nursing experience. When the lack of an academic knowledge base for nursing is taken into consideration, the hypothesis that nurses base a substantial amount of their care upon attitudes and beliefs appears worthy of serious consideration.

Social psychologists have explored the area of attitudes and beliefs and have shown that, while formal logic may be absent at times, we usually tend to show a great deal of consistency and stability in attitudes and beliefs (they are notoriously difficult to change) and also that behaviour is usually consistent with these characteristics. The implication for nursing is that, if practice is based upon attitudes and beliefs, it may tend to lack logic on the one hand, and also be resistant to change on the other. These of course are two characteristics of ritualistic nursing and lead to the suggestion that, as long as nursing bases its practice upon attitudes and beliefs, rather than a sound knowledge base, rituals will continue to be the norm.

If nursing practice is to be more flexible and knowledge-based, ways have to be found of changing attitudes and decreasing dependence upon them as a basis for care. The latter may be achieved by expanding the professional knowledge base of nursing and moving away from training to education.

Attitude change, however, is difficult to achieve but one view worthy of mention briefly is that of the notion of cognitive dissonance theory, which stemmed from the work of Festinger and Carlsmith (1959). The basic notion is that we try and reconcile our actions with beliefs and attitudes and that we feel uncomfortable when this reconciliation is missing. If a person has to do something that is not consistent with his/her beliefs and attitudes, then a state of cognitive dissonance exists – what they think (cognitive) is at odds with what they have to do (dissonance). Experiments carried out by workers such as Festinger and Carlsmith showed that people tend to reconcile this problem by shifting their attitudes and beliefs to harmonize with the new reality of action. In nursing, therefore, we might expect that attitudes could be changed by inducing people to work in different ways. This, of course, requires strong leadership and opens up the whole question of change, which will be looked at in a later chapter.

If attitudes and beliefs are rejected as a suitable knowledge base for practice, what alternative approaches are there to understanding the nature of knowledge? A widely accepted attempt to classify nursing knowledge is that of Carper (1978), who suggested that there are four types of knowledge in nursing: empirics, ethics, aesthetics and personal knowledge. There are other types of knowledge, such as those derived from authority and tradition (Vaughan and Robinson, 1992), and it may be argued that these latter types act as a fifth column, subverting the more academically virtuous notions of Carper.

The term 'empirics' refers to knowledge gained in the scientific, research-based tradition of the natural sciences, such as chemistry and biology. A theory is proposed, a hypothesis deduced from that theory, which is tested by experiment or observation, measurements are made, data are analysed and a probability assigned to the likelihood of the hypothesis being supported or contradicted by the data. This is all the stuff of empirical science and this approach is yielding substantial amounts of knowledge which is of value to nursing.

There is, however, much more to nursing than this effective but limited methodology. The raw matter of nursing is people; therefore notions of moral knowledge become important – hence Carper's reference to ethics. Nurses cannot ignore the moral issues that continually intrude into nursing practice but there are no empirical laws of science that govern topics such as abortion and euthanasia. Ritualistic practice does not permit the nurse to make active decisions, as no decision is necessary to do what we have always done. Moral dilemmas, however, require decisions and consequently if we are to lay claim to being educated professionals, we have to have an understanding of ethics and logical decision-making in the face of moral dilemmas.

Benner's classic work on the development of the expert practitioner (1984) has drawn attention to the intuitive nature of nursing, where the nurse appears to break free from rule-bound practice and intuitively know the right thing to do. Examples of such acts are convincingly documented by Benner. Rew and Berrow (1989) carried out an extensive literature review on the subject of intuition and found that a key theme to emerge was an ability to know something was wrong with a patient before any sign was physically measurable. Critical incident study showed a precognition by the nurse, which was often ignored by the medical staff. Another characteristic was a willingness to try non-traditional methods. These authors conclude by arguing that there is significant evidence to support the validity of intuition as a nursing concept – the art of nursing as proposed by Carper.

Carper's concept of self-knowledge has interesting implications. Nurses are human beings closely interacting with others and as such cannot take themselves out of the clinical equation. The nurse is a key variable in any situation and therefore must be aware of self and how self influences the situation, whether it be the particular mood the nurse is in when greeting a new patient or the nurse's own views on death and mortality while caring for a dying patient. As Vaughan and Robinson point out (1992), the nurse may have studied psychology and try to apply various psychological insights to help the patient, but may also forget that those same insights apply to the nurse. Thus the nurse may forget, feel anxious or use denial as a coping mechanism in exactly the same way as the patient, but does the nurse realize s/he is doing so?

There is something of a paradox within Carper's framework as empirical knowledge is concerned with objective reality, i.e. something exists that is independent of the observer. Different people can see and measure something and get the same results. Empiricism tries to remove observer effects at all costs by strict controls, yet self-knowledge is suggesting the opposite. Self-knowledge underlines the importance of the observer (nurse) as a key actor in any social setting, such as a hospital ward or the patient's home. The situation is not the same without the nurse, and is different for different nurses, therefore objective reality, in which everybody sees the same, is not possible in nursing.

This last point does pose something of a problem in trying to develop a knowledge base for nursing and has been developed by writers such as Campbell and Bunting (1991) and Hagell (1989), who have developed an attack upon empirical orthodoxy from a feminist viewpoint. As nursing develops its own knowledge base, this key question needs urgently to be addressed: do we follow the empirical model of medicine and other sciences, or try and develop a more interactive, subjective approach to knowledge in tune with this feminist critique?

The way forwards

In this introductory chapter we have suggested that there are five major causes of ritualistic practice which may be addressed as follows:

1. Education replacing training as the model for nurse learning.
2. Breaking the gender role stereotyping of nurses as compliant women.
3. Placing clinical research, written in a readily understandable and accessible format, high on nursing's agenda.
4. Admitting that nursing is very stressful and seeking ways of tackling the problems of stress in nursing.
5. Investigating the role that attitudes and beliefs play in shaping nursing practice while studying attitude-change strategies.

There are no easy quick-fix solutions here, but if nursing is to escape from its ritualistic straitjacket, then these are the sort of issues that we must be working on.

Failure to address these questions properly will permit ritualization to continue as part of nursing practice. It will also leave nursing vulnerable to the sort of damage that may be inflicted by false prophets if the profession enthusiastically embraces new ideas before testing them out. Potentially good ideas may become discredited as they have not been implemented in a sound fashion. Alternatively, weak ideas may direct practice in the future, unchallenged and accepted as conventional wisdom by a profession unschooled in the ways of constructive criticism and theory testing. The result, sadly, might be that many of the exciting new ideas that are around today become ossified as new rituals for old.

References

Atkinson R, Atkinson R, Smith E, Hilgard E (1987) *Introduction to Psychology*. New York, Harcourt Brace Jovanovitch.

Benner P (1984) *From Novice to Expert*. New York, Addison Wesley.

Campbell J, Bunting S (1991) Voices and Paradigms. *Advances in Nursing Science* 13: 1–15.

Carper B (1978) Fundamental patterns of knowing in nursing. *Advances in Nursing Science* 1: 13–23.

Chapman G (1983) Ritual and rational actions in hospital. *Journal of Advanced Nursing* 1: 13–20.

Chinn P, Jacobs M (1987) *Theory and Nursing*. St Louis, CV Mosby.

Festinger L, Carlsmith JM (1959) Cognitive consequences of forced compliance. *Journal of Abnormal and Social Psychology* 58: 203–210.

Gerry E (1989) An investigation into the assertive behaviour of trained nurses in general hospital settings. *Journal of Advanced Nursing* 14: 1002–1008.

Graham H (1984) *Women, Health and the Family*. London, Wheatsheaf.

Hagell E (1989) Nursing knowledge: women's knowledge. A sociological perspective. *Journal of Advanced Nursing* **14**: 226–233.

Hayward J (1975) *Information: A Prescription Against Pain*. London, RCN.

Hewstone M, Stroebe W, Codol JP, Stephenson G (1983) *Introduction to Social Psychology*, Oxford, Blackwell.

Kaler S, Levy D, Schall M (1989) Stereotypes of professional roles. *Image, Journal of Nursing Scholarship* **21**: 83–89.

Levy D, Kaler S, Schall M (1988) Stereotypes of professional roles. *Journal of Nursing Education* **21**: 83–89.

Lumby J (1991) Threads of an emerging discipline; praxis, reflection, rhetoric and research. In: Gray G, Pratt R (eds) *Towards a Discipline of Nursing*. Melbourne, Churchill Livingstone.

Meleis A (1991) *Theoretical Nursing, Development and Progress*. Philadelphia, JB Lippincott.

Pitts M, Phillips K (1991) *The Psychology of Health*. London, Routledge.

Rew L, Berrow E (1989) Nurses' intuition: can it coexist with the nursing process? *AORN Journal* **50**: 353–358.

Slater J (1990) Effecting personal effectiveness; assertiveness training for nurses. *Journal of Advanced Nursing* **15**: 337–356.

Smith S (1972) *Nil by Mouth*. London, RCN.

Speedy S (1991) The contribution of feminist research. In: Gray G, Pratt R (eds) *Towards a Discipline of Nursing*. Melbourne, Churchill Livingstone.

University of York Centre for Health Economics (1992) *Skill Mix and the Effectiveness of Nursing Care*. University of York.

Vaughan B, Robinson K (1992) *Knowledge for Nursing Practice*. Oxford, Butterworth-Heinemann.

Walsh M (1991) *Nursing Models in Clinical Practice, The Way Forward*. London, Baillière Tindall.

Walsh M, Ford P (1989) *Nursing Rituals, Research and Rational Actions*. Oxford, Butterworth-Heinemann.

2 Empowering the nurse: a feminist perspective

In the preceding chapter a range of factors were identified which have contributed historically to nursing rituals and which may lead in the future to the introduction of new rituals for old. A common theme running through much of our case is that nurses have been rendered powerless to question practice, to look for different ways of doing things and above all to assert the primacy of caring above other biomedical models. Being powerless is synonymous with being oppressed and one of the principal tenets of feminism is that women are an oppressed group. About 85% of nurses also happen to be women. It is hard to ignore making a linkage between these two statements and, in addressing the issue of empowerment, feminist perspectives therefore deserve our immediate attention.

The concept of empowerment has appeared in the nursing literature within the last few years, applied mostly to empowering patients. However, some writers have taken this concept further and applied it to nursing itself and it is this approach, in the context of what empowerment of nursing may achieve, that will form the theme of this chapter.

The issues of oppression and empowerment are central to liberating nursing from ritualistic practice and therefore allowing nurses the chance to grow and express themselves to their full potential. As long as nursing accepts its subservient role to medicine and the new managerialism of the post-1990 NHS, and as long as we are willing to accept new concepts uncritically as things which have to be implemented because an expert says this is the way forwards, then rituals will persist at the expense of caring. If a lack of power is one of the main causes of ritualistic practice, then perhaps the empowerment of nursing is the logical way forwards.

Empowerment is a difficult concept to define as it is very subjective in nature – one person's empowerment may be another's subversion, for example. The definition offered by Mason *et al.* (1991) however accords well with the consensus that may be derived from reading the literature. These authors suggest that empowerment is concerned with the equitable distribution of power so that people may participate fully in actions and decision-making. From this notion flows the idea that connections between self and others are essential so that all may recognize their strengths and abilities. Self- and group awareness are therefore key concepts if nursing is to move away from ritualistic practice and the domination of outside groups.

Within the literature of empowerment there is an innovative way of looking at the concept of power which is derived from feminist thinking and characterized by the writings of Miller (1976), who suggests that men and women see power differently. Men see it as a finite and limited resource to be competed over with a view to winning as large a portion as possible which is then to be guarded, extended if possible and used over others. This empire-building model will be very familiar to many nurses. Women, however, see power as something to be shared within a context of respect for others, equality and consensus. It is this latter view of power that feminist writers have urged nurses, as a predominantly female group, to work with in pursuit of empowerment.

Ironically, this is precisely the opposite trend to the path being followed by the NHS under the ideological directive of the Conservative government. Consensus management was scrapped in 1985 with the Griffiths Report and the introduction of general management, while subsequently reform of the NHS has been constructed around simple market forces.

Within the male view of power, it is easy to see how ritualistic practice develops as staff are seen as subordinates whose job is to follow orders. Nursing's historical origins go a long way to explaining why, despite nursing being predominantly female, this hierarchical male model predominates. Within the feminist view, however, there is room for debate and alternative points of view which are positively encouraged. Such an approach may well lead to a range of different solutions to problems rather than nursing by the procedure manual.

Before exploring this feminist view of empowerment further, it is necessary to look at the position of nurses today and the suggestion that nurses constitute an oppressed group. There can be little doubt today that many nurses feel they lack power and that they are continually being asked to do more with less resources. Seccombe and Ball (1992) have shown that there is widespread dissatisfaction amongst nurses with the care they are able to give and that this is closely correlated with excessive workloads and inadequate staffing levels. Dissatisfaction was much more pronounced amongst nurses within the NHS who were far more negative than those outside. This study also found that, while nurses liked their work, they were much less happy with the state of nursing itself.

The increasing stresses being placed upon staff are revealed in the staff-side evidence to the Pay Review Body (Nursing and Midwifery Staff's Negotiating Council, 1992), which shows that more patients at a higher level of dependence are being treated than ever before. For example, between 1987 and 1991 there was a 9% increase in the level of activity within the NHS with a forecast rise of 3.7% in the year 1991–1992. During this period, however, the number of nursing staff has remained constant, although there has been a substantial rise in administrative staff (between 1980 and 1990 administrative staff rose by 20% according to data cited by the staff side). The picture that emerges from reports such as these mentioned here is of a nurse workforce which is under ever-increasing pressure and which is showing all the tell-tale signs of declining morale and a sense of powerlessness.

Nurses might sometimes wonder if anybody is listening to their voices within the corridors of power. However assiduously organizations such as the Royal College of Nursing may work to lobby on behalf of nurses, the changes keep coming thick and fast. The male view of power is in the ascendency as the predominantly male senior managers hang on to their power and enthusiastically wield it over others with little or no thought of heeding other points of view or of sharing their control. Nobody seems to want to know what nurses think.

The NHS has been carved up into Trusts, without any evidence to suggest this will change things for the better; worrying rumours persist about the future of the Pay Review Body; employers write gagging clauses into contracts to prevent nurses speaking out about patient conditions, whilst major nursing redundancies are looming on the horizon. The skill-mix and reprofiling exercises currently being carried out are suspected of merely being an exercise to justify substantial reductions in the numbers of qualified staff employed in care delivery. The economic hardships of the early 1990s are making an increasing number of nurses the sole breadwinner within their families as unemployment continues to take its toll. When it is so easy to paint such a gloomy picture as this, it is small wonder that many nurses do feel powerless and decide that the best thing to do is to keep your head down, go along with the system, don't rock the boat and survive.

Another factor which has to be considered in painting this picture of oppression is the notion that knowledge is power. As we argued in the first chapter, a serious problem for nursing has been its historical lack of a sound academic foundation. The result has been in the past the appearance of prejudice, attitudes and beliefs on the one hand, dressed up as nursing wisdom, while on the other hand the larder of biomedicine has been raided to provide some sort of credible knowledge base for nursing. Recent work is addressing this problem as a matter of urgency; however the lack of a serious academic foundation for nursing has hindered its development as a profession and led to the medical view of the nurse sometimes resembling that of a serf.

There is ample evidence therefore to consider nurses today as an oppressed group, whether it be by virtue of gender, government policy, lack of a perceived academic base or the power struggle within the NHS. Nurses should not give in to a discourse of despair, however, as it is possible to reclaim nursing for nurses and in the process construct a new nursing free from ritualistic practice. This chapter began with the notion of empowerment and it is there we must return to examine some feminist perspectives that may assist nurses to reclaim nursing.

Feminism is a general term that embraces a wide range of views about women's place in society, although these positions are linked by the common theme that women are an oppressed group within a male-directed society which may be described as a patriarchy.

Speedy (1991) has summarized the different schools of feminist thought into four broad categories, the first of which, cultural feminism, holds that liberation for women cannot occur in a patriarchal culture but instead it requires the growth of a matriarchal culture before women can genuinely be free. This of course begs the question of what happens to men in such a matriarchal culture? Do they in their turn become an oppressed group? A less extreme position is taken by liberal feminists who argue that women can achieve liberation within the system. There is room in their view for change from within by education and reform. Socialist feminism links the oppression of women to class and racial oppression and sees this as part of capitalist exploitation of the workforce. Finally, radical feminism holds that the exploitation of women by men is the most profound and ingrained form of oppression in the human race, seeing it almost in the same light as the doctrine of original sin.

It is worth acknowledging that there is this range of views within the feminist movement and also that these positions are only simplifications of a very complex reality. Entering into a discussion about the merits of the different positions, especially with regard to nursing, would be an interesting debate. The resolution of such a debate may take much time and energy; the problem of freeing and empowering nursing, however, is immediate. It is worth noting in regard to cultural feminism that, if 85% of nurses are women, is this not a matriarchal society? Cultural feminism therefore has to deal with an apparent paradox. Failure to achieve liberation within nursing therefore suggests that the control of the outside, patriarchal society overrides nursing's own ability to control itself, or more subtly, perhaps nurses have adopted the ways of the oppressor and behaved in male ways towards their predominantly female colleagues.

Briefly commenting on the other perspectives, it should be noted that the socialist view is consistent with the low rates of pay that are characteristic of nurses worldwide. Nurses are seen as cheap labour. The liberal view offers the best chance of improving nurses' lot, as it suggests that change can occur within the system with the minimum of turbulence, but the radical view suggests that change is going to be extremely difficult.

An essential step in empowerment is the realization by nurses that they are subordinated within the health-care system to others in a way that can be viewed as oppression. Such consciousness-raising is a key component of feminism. Feminist nurses such as Speedy (1991) argue that, while caring is fundamental to nursing, the view that it is naturally feminine and unique to nursing will do nurses great harm as it will devalue women and nurses, unless looked at in conjunction with the issues of power relations within the NHS and society in general. Men can care as well as women whilst nurses are not the only people who can care for others. The view that female nurses are naturally suited to provide care while men tell them what to do should be anathema to all nurses and only by exposing this as the dangerous myth that it is will nursing enable itself to develop its practice in a valued and creative way.

Smith (1988) talked of 'doing feminism' as challenging institutional power structures and relationships, challenging domination within nursing and, in the process, offering the opportunity of transforming health care in such a way that nurses and women become active participants in their own futures. Such an approach would also free nursing practice from the burden of ritual and tradition. It should also try and take men along with it wherever possible, whether they are nurses or not.

These views are echoed by Vidovich (1990), who has argued for a feminist critique of the traditional male values that permeate the health-care system in her native Australia in order that the value of caring may achieve its full recognition instead of being ridiculed by some, as at present. The UK experience is more akin to being patronized, at least in public, although in private caring may receive its share of ridicule also. The nurse's view on the ward round may still be dismissed as unimportant, sometimes with thinly veiled irritation at this intrusion of a caring perspective into the medical domain.

The relevance of her views to nursing is underlined in Vidovich's view by the fact that, while women have broken into many traditional male bastions and occupy positions that were unthinkable a generation ago, the energy expended in doing so has led to the neglect by women of areas that have been traditionally their domain, such as nursing. Does this explain the paradox hinted at earlier, that despite nursing being a matriarchy, women still feel they are an oppressed group within nursing? Vidovich characterizes the operation of the health service in Australia as structured misogyny: is there any evidence to suggest that this phrase might not also apply to the UK?

The links between nursing, feminism and empowerment are spelt out bluntly by Krieger (1991), who argues that the key aspect of a feminist education is empowerment and then goes on to criticize nursing education for its lack of empowerment. Rather, it produces students who are essentially conformist, do not participate actively in their education and eventually are destined to become cannon-fodder for the big hospitals where they will simply do what they are told. This is a transatlantic view of nursing education, but it has echoes that reverberate still in the UK. If, in 1992, a group of students can still be disciplined for 'being insolent' in complaining about low standards of care, some educationalists at least have a case to answer. The issue of training rather than education has already been raised as contributing towards ritualistic nursing. Krieger urges nurse educators to adopt feminist strategies which will make the classroom a supportive place where students can take risks, where cooperation and collaboration are the norm and competition and destructive criticism are discouraged.

Feminists argue that women have patterns of knowing that are different from the empirical tradition that dominates male-fashioned science. However, while empirical knowledge is necessary for nursing practice, so too are these other forms of knowing and Krieger argues that for nurses to regain the essence of nursing and thus enhance the quality of care, they need, as women, to rethink their position in society and address these issues. If this analysis is correct – that knowledge depends upon the knower and therefore women know things differently from men – nursing education has to facilitate this process of highlighting the value of women's knowledge.

This still leaves the problem of the 10–15% of UK nurses who are men, however. Do they know nursing differently from their female colleagues? If the answer is yes, then nursing needs to reconcile these different types of knowing. In examining nursing from the feminist perspective, it has to be remembered that many of the writers being considered here are either American or Australian; there are significantly fewer men in nursing in these countries than in the UK. Generalizations about nursing being a female occupation need to be tempered with the fact that UK nursing has a significant minority of men. Is it impossible to suggest that men in nursing, given an appropriate education, could come to know nursing at least in part as women know nursing? Some men at least are capable of seeing another person's point of view (an essential skill for nurses of either gender), so why should not men be capable of seeing nursing from another perspective, even if they have not the lived experience of being a woman? Ethical and personal knowledge, together with intuition and the common-sense knowledge of 'knowing in doing', make up the other dimensions of nursing knowledge and should be accessible to men as well as women.

The traditional view of education has been the passing-on of knowledge. If nursing education is simply about empirical facts and therefore students are treated as passive receptacles of knowledge, just empty vessels to be filled up with facts, argues Krieger, they will never learn to learn for themselves. Students will fail to develop as independent thinkers and fall naturally into the handmaiden stereotype. This critical view of education is derived from the analysis of Freire (1970), who argues passionately for the active involvement of students in the learning process if education is not to become a means of social control, which has the hidden agenda of ensuring students conform to the system when qualified. Paolo Freire's work as a radical educationalist will be discussed in more depth in the next chapter but he has many powerful ideas about empowerment which, as we shall see, are very relevant to nurses today. There is much more to nursing education than simply passing on facts or empirical knowledge, and this applies equally in the clinical area and the classroom, to ward staff and to nurse teachers.

An empowering education could permit nurses to promote caring to a position of primacy and make it not just a nursing issue but a health-care issue. In this way it becomes part of the general health-care agenda and not just a women's issue or a nurse's issue, and as such has to be addressed by all concerned within the health service. As long as caring is not seen in this way, the male-dominated management élite will continue to focus on the medically driven, high-tech, high-cost budget items and medical science will continue to dominate the agenda at the expense of undervalued caring. The prime concern of most nurses – caring – will continue to be low down the agenda amongst 'any other business'.

Set a thief to catch a thief is an old adage. Can nursing put caring on to the health agenda, at least on a par with medicine, by adopting the ways of the medical profession? Should women try and achieve results by adopting the methods of men, such as, for example, Mrs Thatcher in her ruthless pursuit of political power? This question is put by Mason *et al.* (1991), who argue that nursing would be making a mistake if it did. In their view nursing should not adopt the values of the power élite nor play the game by their rules. Nursing should first value itself and then seek to integrate nursing issues into the larger health field, as outlined above.

It is not easy to go on to a basketball court and try to play netball, which by analogy is what these authors seem to be suggesting. However, the notion of improving nursing's self-esteem is worth following, but alongside that, nursing has to demonstrate its value to others. Mason *et al.* are arguing for nursing to become fully involved in the political process if it is to advance the values of caring into the mainstream of health. Nursing in the past has not been very successful in this enterprise, hence its subordinated position, which is the key to understanding the perpetuation of routinized and unthinking patterns of care.

Various authors have argued that nursing does not value itself enough, and without this self-esteem, how can nurses expect others to value them and their contribution to health, except in the patronizing way that we are all familiar with every time a Secretary of State, for example, addresses a major conference, such as the Royal College of Nursing annual congress? Jenny (1990), for example, argues that to the patient, nobody is more important in the health-care team than the nurse, so why do nurses doubt themselves so much? She answers her own question by pointing to the way nursing has in the past failed to differentiate itself from medicine, the lack of an academic base of nursing knowledge, lack of professional unity and the lack of appreciation of the real power that nurses do have. Jenny, like many other authors, then goes on to reinforce the argument that nurses as women are suppressed by men as part of the wider gender inequality in society, citing research by people such as Lasky (1983), which shows that women tend to have lower self-esteem than men anyway. Nurses need to work on their self-concept and self-esteem if they are to achieve the autonomy to practise that is essential for professional care.

Western society has had a deep prejudice against women being involved in the political process. They have been considered lacking in rationality and too emotional for effective politics. It is no coincidence that, while the medical profession has traditionally been well-represented in the House of Commons, that august body still awaits its first nurse member.

If prejudice has tied one arm behind nursing's back, nursing has, according to Mason *et al.*, tied its other arm itself by perpetuating the wider inequalities of society within the profession and also holding on to views that see political activity as unprofessional and even unfeminine. The way enrolled nurses have been treated in the UK is a classic example of Mason's criticisms, whilst the serious over-representation of black nurses in the nursing auxiliary and enrolled nurse grades suggests the existence of institutional racism within nursing. British nursing is guilty of perpetuating social inequalities within its ranks; this results in an acceptance of subordination as a normal state of affairs. Routinized care, carried out with little thought and question, is the expected result where hierarchies and inequalities are predominant and, sadly, this has been one of the hallmarks of nursing since Nightingale's time. A more egalitarian approach is badly needed within nursing if nurses are to be free to question and challenge practice.

The values of caring are at odds with overriding male conventional wisdom and goals according to feminists, yet is is males who control the health-care system. Feminists concentrate on processes involving collaboration, equality and collectivity; NHS managers are only concerned with outcomes and efficiency. This is a major challenge facing nursing today as the pressure is increasing all the time on ward and community staff to produce results, improve throughput and cut costs. Not only are such pressures at odds with feminist thinking – they also prohibit empowerment of nursing as decisions have to be made quickly, there is no time for sharing and consensus became a dirty word with the introduction of general management in the aftermath of the Griffiths Report. Trying to practise under such pressures leaves the nurse with little scope for experimentation and innovation, the routine triumphs over originality which in turn becomes a luxury disqualified by managerial edict. There simply is not time to think.

Nursing as a result becomes locked into a vicious circle of surviving, somehow getting the work done, and as a consequence fails to value itself even further. Nurses feel despondent because they know the care they are giving falls below their own standards. This issue of nurses' self-perceptions has been explored by Morrison (1989), who carried out an in-depth questionnaire study on 25 Sisters and charge nurses in a range of general and psychiatric nursing areas. The study could be summarized as asking the staff to describe their ideal self-image as nurses and then comparing themselves with that ideal view. The results showed that there were very substantial differences for most of the nurses who took part. The author admits that there were procedural difficulties which could have introduced bias, in that asking individuals to describe an ideal and then compare themselves with it is almost inviting them to acknowledge discrepancies.

Morrison feels, however, that despite this difficulty his findings still have validity. He found that nurses could not live up to their ideal levels of performance and therefore role discrepancies might commonly be experienced by nurses. The fact that they fall short of their ideals may therefore be seen as a source of personal conflict and have adverse effects upon practice. Three possible reasons are advanced to explain why nurses feel they fall short of what they should be achieving, the most interesting of which is that the nurse may have a different value system to that of the organization. While the nurse may value caring and interpersonal skills, the organization values technical, task-focused skills and so the nurse feels s/he has to achieve the goal of 'getting the work done' and displaying high-tech skills, rather than caring in the fullest sense of the word. Additionally, the lack of self-esteem may stem from setting goals that are unrealistically high and an inadequate knowledge base.

Although the main theme that emerged was one of nurses rating themselves below the ideal, a subplot also emerged in that half the nurses consistently downrated the ideal self on key aspects of the caring role. This was explained as a defence against the personal costs to the carer of aiming too high – in other words, the cost of aiming so high would be to leave the nurse emotionally and physically drained. This is an issue that we will return to in Chapter 6, namely, setting standards can be detrimental if they are set too high, as they may then lead to exhaustion and a sense of failure and underachievement.

This particular study therefore shows that within the UK there is evidence that nurses do underestimate themselves and have a low self-esteem. It should be noted, though, that it is only one study and needs replicating, perhaps with two different matched groups. In this way, the first group could be used to measure the ideal self while a well-matched second group could give actual self-ratings on the same aspects of nursing. This would avoid the problem encountered in Morrison's study of asking people to state an ideal and compare themselves against it, which could lead to biased results.

If nurses feel they must get the work done and feel guilty if they do not achieve a certain list of tasks, they will suffer a lowering of self-esteem which, as we have seen, is one of the reasons for nursing's subordinate status. Additionally, depersonalized and routinized conveyor-belt nursing will result, and with it the propagation into the future of unthinking, ritualistic nursing practice.

That such feelings of inadequacy exist, and that they may be tackled by an empowering approach to education, has been shown by the work of Lutz *et al.* (1991). This team of educators set themselves the task of designing a course that would lead to students who were assertive, creative, inquiring, curious and caring. Their basic strategy was one of empowerment and the tactics they deployed consisted of student-led seminars alongside close liaison with clinical staff. The principles of empowerment described earlier were implemented from a feminist perspective within groups. Students were encouraged to collaborate and take risks while feeling safe; consensus rather than competition was encouraged.

Early on, students expressed frustration due to continual pressure from staff to have tasks done by certain times and the feeling that students were rated as good if they got the jobs done by coffee- or lunch-time. Students admitted rarely talking to patients as they focused on tasks instead. Nursing care was equated with completing tasks, with the result that procedures became the ends of nursing care rather than one of the means by which nursing care was carried out. This picture is instantly recognizable as being associated with ritualistic nursing and could have been taken directly from the account given by Walsh and Ford (1989) in their original discussion of rituals in nursing.

It is encouraging, however, that following the involvement of students, teachers and staff working together in this series of empowering seminars, changes occurred. Students felt able to talk about patients with ward staff; they were able to experiment and take risks (within obvious limits, of course): they tried to do things differently and moved away from ward routines towards a more flexible patient-centred approach. Education staff came to the interesting conclusion that when trust and the desire to share real nursing experiences are present, students and teachers can empower each other to behave in new ways which help students find new meanings in, and creative ways of, practising professional nursing. The two key words here are *trust* and *sharing*, which are the very embodiment of empowerment and very distant from the traditional (male) view of power relationships.

The other lesson to be learnt is that teachers must work with ward staff; education cannot occur in a vacuum, nor is it confined to pre-registration students. By working with the ward staff in this way, not only did the teachers empower the students to develop a creative and questioning approach to care but they also had a similar effect upon the ward staff. Empowerment programmes may also be directed at qualified staff; they are not the prerogative of students. Brooks and Pares (1990) provide a vivid account of such work as part of a professional development programme. The outcome was very favourably evaluated by the nurses who took part, as they stated how, starting as individuals, they had come together as a group who now felt able to influence and change things about the workplace and also in their home lives. Interestingly, they felt more positive about the hospital management as they felt valued by management as a result of such courses being provided. It is unrealistic to expect students to practise in an empowered and creative way unless the ward staff have a similar philosophy.

In the introduction to this chapter, it was stated that the discussion on empowerment would largely be confined to nurses rather than patients. It is worth reminding ourselves at this stage, however, that empowering the patient also involves nursing in empowering itself. This view is supported by the work of Gibson (1991), who carried out an in-depth review of the literature on patient empowerment. In her view, empowerment consists of helping people assert control over their lives and is a composite of attributes that relate to the patient, the nurse and both jointly. The precursor for empowerment is that people must develop a critical awareness of the root causes of their problems and then be ready to act on this awareness – this comment applies equally to patients and nurses.

According to Gibson, empowerment is a double-edged sword for, if nurses are to campaign for empowerment of nursing, they must also campaign for empowerment of the patient and recognize that the patient is an equal partner in the health-care team. Just as nurses need to trust each other and collaborate as equals, so too must they trust the patient and let go of their traditional power as the health professional who knows best. It is inconsistent to advocate empowerment and all that goes with it for nurses if we do not extend this concept to patients. This involves a radical shift in thinking for all health professionals.

Empowerment should produce a sense of control and self-determination, growth, a sense of connectedness and cooperation with others and a sense of well-being. These postulated outcomes see empowerment as an independent variable. Turning the question around the other way and asking what will lead to empowerment sees the concept as a dependent variable. Answers might be giving information to facilitate participation in decision-making and providing support, collaboration and education. By looking at the concept in this way Gibson gives some useful clues in checking whether empowerment is really taking place in practice.

The giving of information in itself, however, is not empowering. Management often sees consultation as telling people what is going to happen, inviting their comments and carrying on with preset plans regardless. Doctors and managers are often accused of not giving information to nurses: we should therefore not merely be grateful when they do, but say that this is not enough. Malin and Teasdale (1991) have produced some interesting case-study research to show that empowerment of patients (and therefore by analogy, of nurses) is not just about giving information, as this in itself may not offer the opportunity for control that is an essential characteristic of empowerment.

Giving information gives predictability – the patient or nurse knows what will happen, but that in itself is not empowering. Telling the patient what will happen before and after an operation informs the patient and allows him or her to predict what will happen so things do not come as a surprise, but it does not in itself allow that person any control over the type of operation or levels of post-operative analgesia, for example. Telling nurses that primary nursing is going to be introduced on their ward or that shift patterns are going to be changed allows them to predict what will happen to some extent, but in itself does not give the nursing staff any control or sense of ownership of the new system. Management should therefore be aware that giving information is not enough; empowerment involves fully engaging staff and allowing them to have equal control of the professional issues involved.

In this chapter we have argued that if nurses are to be able to change how they practise in such a way that they can be creative and innovative, they need to value themselves, to share with each other and work in a spirit of collaboration and, above all, to reclaim nursing as the prerogative of nurses, with patients as equal partners. Such goals are about empowerment and consistent with a feminist approach, which rejects the notion of power that is jealously guarded by the few to be wielded over the many.

When nurses feel able to do things differently, try out ideas without fear of failure, work together as members of a team of equals with each other rather than in the hierarchical structures that still bedevil nursing today, then routinized, ritualistic nursing will at last begin to fade from the scene. When nurses no longer do what they are told, but rather what in their professional judgement they think is right, nursing will be in a position to avoid having new rituals imposed upon itself from the medico-management élite and also from within its own ranks. Is this pie in the sky? We suggest not, as a feminist approach to nursing does contain worthwhile and new ideas which can guide nursing forwards and away from a past dominated by traditional male values which have served only to oppress nurses and nursing.

One final word of caution, however: empowerment and self-assertion classes must be sensitive to the gender of those participating. Assertive behaviour is stereotypically seen as normal in men but lacking in women. Kilkus (1990) suggests that as the concept of assertiveness was, like so many others, defined originally by men, it had its definition constructed in such a way as to exclude women. Men therefore were seeking to devalue the perceptions and experiences of women. Assertiveness training offers a route by which women can make their voices heard again, but that training should not be along the lines that are normally defined as assertive, for this definition is gender-sensitive. Training women in assertiveness by the male rule-book only disadvantages women further; rather, assertiveness training for women which emphasizes women's perceptions is what is required.

As Kilkus points out, nurses have had to contend with a long history of subordination and being seen as a passive and docile group who will always do what they are told. Assertiveness, however, can offer nurses the chance to construct a new model of caring based on respect for others, honesty and trust – aspects which are sometimes lacking from the conventional models of medically-driven care that we see around us. An empowered nursing profession, rejecting traditional male models of power, can establish, in Benner and Wrubel's words (1989), 'the primacy of caring'.

References

Benner P, Wrubel J (1989) *The Primacy of Caring*. Menlo Pk Ca, Addison-Wesley.

Brooks S, Pares J (1990) Empowering nurses: a professional development programme. *The Lamp* November, 23–27.

Freire P (1970) *Pedagogy of the Oppressed*. New York, Seabury Press.

Freire P (1972) *The Pedagogy of the Oppressed*. Ramos B (translator). London, Pelican.

Gibson C (1991) A concept analysis of empowerment. *Journal of Advanced Nursing* **16**: 354–361.

Griffiths R (1985) *Inquiry into NHS Management*. London, Department of Health.

Jenny J (1990) Self esteem: a problem for nurses. *Canadian Nurse* November, 19–21.

Kilkus S (1990) Self-assertion and nurses: a different voice. *Nursing Outlook* May/June, 143–145.

Krieger S (1991) Nursing education and feminism. *Canadian Nurse* September, 30–32.

Lasky E (1983) Self-esteem, achievement and the female experience. In: Muff J (ed) *Socialisation, Sexism and Stereotyping: Women's Issues in Nursing*. St. Louis, CV Mosby.

Lutz M, Petrovic K, Miller C (1991) The empowering nature of educative learning. *Journal of Nursing Education* 30: 40–42.

Malin N, Teasdale K (1991) Caring versus empowerment: considerations for nursing practice. *Journal of Advanced Nursing* 16: 657–662.

Mason D, Backer B, Georges A (1991) Towards a feminist model for the empowerment of nurses. *Image, Journal of Nursing Scholarship* 23: 72–77.

Miller JB (1976) *Towards a New Psychology for Women*. Boston, Beacon.

Nursing and Midwifery Staff's Negotiating Council (1992) *Evidence to Review Body for Nursing Staff*. London.

Morrison P (1989) Nursing and caring: a personal self-construct theory of some nurses' perceptions. *Journal of Advanced Nursing* 14: 421–426.

Seccombe I, Ball J (1992) *Motivation, Morals and Mobility*. IMS Report 233. London, Institute of Manpower Studies, Royal College of Nursing.

Smith S (1988) A feminist analysis of constructs of health. Conference Proceedings. *Caring and Nursing: Exploration in the Feminist Perspectives*. Denver.

Speedy S (1991) The contribution of feminist research. In: Gray G, Pratt R (eds) *Towards a Discipline of Nursing*. Edinburgh, Churchill Livingstone.

Vidovich, M (1990) The tragic tale of the feminist nurse. *Australian Nurses' Journal* 20: 12–14.

Walsh M, Ford P (1989) *Nursing Rituals: Research and Rational Action*. Oxford, Butterworth-Heinemann.

3 Empowerment, nursing and clinical practice

If we are to reclaim and regenerate nursing, we must look at our profession with a fresh sense of vision and from new points of view. Feminism is only one such standpoint from which the field of nursing may be viewed. In this chapter we will look at another – the notion of critical social theory, particularly as advocated by one of the early leaders of the liberation theology movement, Paolo Freire, and see that his views have striking relevance for nursing, so much so that we might usefully talk of empowerment as liberation nursing. When the writings of authors such as Schon (1983) and Benner (1984) are taken together with these new perspectives, we contend that it is indeed possible for nurses to reclaim nursing and in the process avoid a future that mirrors our ritualistic past.

The touchstone for any analysis of oppression has usually been the writings of Karl Marx. However, with the delicious irony that history sometimes reserves for the famous, Marxist–Leninist ideology has been, in the words of one of its early leaders, Trotsky, 'consigned to the dustbin of history', at least for the time being! The notion that groups oppress other groups on the basis of class is simplistic anyway as it ignores factors such as race, gender and age, the 'isms' of current sociological thought.

For a more relevant view of the problems facing nursing today, the work of critical social theorists such Paulo Freire offers a more fruitful approach. Freire's early work (1970) was born of his experiences working in the field of adult education in Brazil where he became aware of the use of education as a double-edged sword that could, in the hands of one group of people, enforce oppression, while in the hands of the oppressed themselves, could be used for empowerment and escape from oppression. Education therefore offers a way forwards, but how?

The starting point might be an assertion by Grioux (1985), who argues that history is never foreclosed. People may be limited by constraints, but those constraints are only made by humans and as such are subject to challenge by humans. In other words, nursing may be constrained by outside forces but these are derived from ordinary human beings and as such are subject to challenge by nurses. The definitive book on the history of nursing can never be written because, unlike an accountant's ledger, it can never be closed as there is no end to history. Nursing has evolved a long way since Nightingale, but it can go on changing and evolving and, if we take a long-term view beyond the doom and gloom of the present, there really is hope in the future. History is not foreclosed with a definite ending that is inevitable; it can be changed by the actions of nurses today, tomorrow and the day after.

The reader may wonder what is the relevance of a Third World educationalist to nursing in the UK. First, it has to be said that Freire has lived and written about education and power in both the USA and elsewhere, not just Latin America. More to the point, however, is Freire's views (1985) on what happens when one society dominates another: his views have a remarkable resonance with the position of nurses with regard to doctors. In Freire's view, the dominated group (nurses) absorb the cultural myths of the dominators (doctors) together with their values and lifestyles; they have their structures and infrastructures shaped by the dominators but are without their strength and resources. The result of this is that the dominated group cannot cope with challenge and so imposes rigid and inflexible structures upon its members while it is constructed as a silent society. It has no authentic voice of its own – only an echo of the dominator's society, the society that speaks while the dominated listens. Within the dominated society this silence is repeated towards its own as they are silenced should they speak out of turn.

This powerful analysis of oppressed societies worldwide should be recognizable to nurses. Traditionally, nurses have had a parallel hierarchy to doctors, reinforced by uniforms and various rituals, including the, at times, inhumane and humiliating treatment of juniors. When doctors have taught nurses, set exam papers, sat on nursing's ruling bodies, written nursing textbooks that consisted of watered-down medical knowledge that doctors thought fit for nurses to know, and until very recently interviewed nurses for nursing posts, it is small wonder that nurses absorbed many medical values and aspects of lifestyle. Things are changing undoubtedly but nurses still use medical jargon extensively, even down to the North American practice of defining patient problems as 'nursing diagnoses'. Stethoscopes are casually slung across the back of the shoulders or draped around the neck by nurses in imitation of the medical style, while off duty, parties in the doctor's mess remain attractive to many nurses. In themselves, perhaps none of these things matter, except to show that nursing is still caught up within the medical frame of reference. Perhaps it is unrealistic to expect it to be otherwise given the nature of nursing and medicine, but that does not detract from Freire's analysis as a valid explanation of much nursing behaviour.

That nursing lacks the strength and resources of medicine is self-evident, leading to the traditional imposition of authoritarian rule by ward sisters of yore, which still persists in some wards today. Ritualistic patterns of nursing are born of an inflexible, rigid approach which, according to Freire, characterizes the oppressed. Fear of a student asking a question that the person in authority cannot answer, or of a staff nurse wanting to do things differently and in the process undermining the authority of the Sister, is typical of a person holding authority under false pretences as he or she lacks the knowledge base to legitimize that authority. Questions are silenced, strangled in the inquirer's throat by Sister's glare. Modern NHS management stands guilty of the charge that it cannot tolerate nurses who question and blow the whistle on bad practice: nurses are silenced by gagging clauses in their contracts. Some, at least, of the macho managers of today are showing traits that are characteristic of oppressors.

Ritualistic behaviour and authoritarian resistance to change may therefore be seen as a product of the inevitable stresses and strains set up in a situation where one group of people holds power which they are determined to keep at the expense of another subordinate group. This male view contrasts with the feminist perception of power as being about consensus and sharing, which suggests that the feminist point of view might help nursing away from ritualistic behaviour as nurses are encouraged to collaborate rather than follow orders.

There are other subtle means by which the controlling group in a society can keep their power at the expense of subordinate groups. Giroux (1985) has suggested that education may be used as a means of social control. He summarizes the arguments of many radical critics by pointing out that the notion that education is about letting students explore their own abilities and extend their knowledge in an open and free environment is open to abuse. He argues that education may be used to propagate the culture, values and norms of those in control within a society in such a way that alternative views are suppressed: education is therefore a means of social control. Knowledge is selectively passed on in a way that reflects a certain world view, a pattern of social relations and ways of thinking and behaving. Education may not be ideologically neutral but constructed in such a way as to maintain the status quo with regard to power and control.

A brief review of the history of nurse education sees the dominance of the medical profession being reinforced by traditional nurse tutors throughout most of the last 100 years. The authors of this book received much of their nurse training from doctors and were, for example, required to stand when a doctor entered a classroom to lecture and also expected to address doctors as 'sir'. As students, we learned in this way that doctors were valued above nurses. It is not difficult to see how education may be used to propagate the status quo in terms of social relations and power structures.

In Chapter 1, traditional nurse training was blamed for the propagation of many rituals and myths. It is some comfort therefore to see this as only part of a much wider social phenomenon affecting education in general. The move towards greater professional autonomy in nursing during the last 20 years has started to remove some of these controls and the accelerating progress towards higher education will hasten the process. Nurse educators still need, however, to look at themselves in the mirror and ask to what extent is the educational experience they offer students ideologically neutral? Only by such self-evaluation can we be sure that we do not continue to propagate ideas and messages that are contrary to the ethos of professional autonomy, which is essential if we are to move away from ritualistic practice.

A key concept within this field is that education should be more than the simple transference of knowledge which describes reality (as seen by those in authority), for this will only lead to the political illiteracy of the student and prevent the development of a critical consciousness. Nurses have in the past been criticized for their political naïvety, which is not surprising in the light of this analysis. Freire believes that students are not just empty vessels to be filled up with facts, yet dominating education strives to achieve just that goal by taming and domesticating students' critical faculties. This leads to the meek acceptance of what is taught as automatically correct and consequently the development of an uncritical practitioner. The road to rituals is paved with the passive acceptance of 'facts' rather than challenging assertions, and copious note-taking rather than critical thought.

Education must overcome this domesticizing tendency, which fills the student's head with safe facts and conventional wisdom, leading to the atrophy of critical faculties. Conscientization is a word much used in critical social theory; it means to participate critically in a transforming act. Defined in such a way, it has great significance in nursing for educators and clinical nurses alike. They must strive to promote recognition that the world of nursing practice is something dynamic and full of change rather than a static backwater. This is particularly true in post-registration education where initiatives such as the English Nursing Board's Higher Award must produce practitioners who can challenge and change the system rather than sponges who can only absorb more facts.

Conscientization is also said to bring about the removal of cultural myths that serve to confuse people's awareness of reality. Nursing has plenty of cultural myths that do indeed confuse reality. If nurses with critical awareness and enquiring minds engage themselves in day-to-day clinical practice, transforming that practice by a process of reflection and innovation, then it seems likely that many of our cultural myths will be challenged and displaced. Task-oriented care may finally be displaced by patient-centred care and the devaluing myth that nursing is just about a simple collection of tasks that anybody can do will be displaced by the reality of individualized, holistic care, clarifying the issue of professional accountability in the process. This process of changing by doing is sometimes known as praxis and offers nursing an exciting avenue of potential growth away from the fragmented, task-focused approach that some still advocate.

A key observation made by Freire is that power may be used in such a way that subordinate groups actively but unknowingly participate in their own subordination. He points out that domination is more than the obvious enforcement agencies of control (disciplinary committees, contracts, etc.). Rather, it is about the way ideology combines with power structures and also technology to produce types of knowledge, patterns of relation-ships and other cultural manifestations that operate actively to silence people. The subordinate group learns to internalize its subordination and it becomes a part of their collective personality – almost a collective need born perhaps of the desire for security.

In this way, the subordinate group participates in its own subordination.

In nursing we have had to work with a male, medical-dominated ideology and power structures that gave power to doctors and latterly to the new breed of managers. We are having to come to terms with the new ideologies of market forces determining whether a hospital stays open or not rather than patient need, and the notion that managers have the power to close hospitals regardless of patient need or the views of the professional staff who work within them, including doctors.

Technology has given doctors an enormous range of options for the practice of medical science yet each intervention, whether it be the development of ventilatory support systems, new surgical interventions that were previously impossible or new drugs, always seems to produce the same thing – a live patient in need of ever more intensive nursing care, dependent upon more and more sophisticated medical science.

The ingredients of power, ideology and technology are all present. What evidence is there, however, that they produce subordination and hence ritualistic practice? There is no doubt that the types of knowledge that abound in nursing are medically driven, although less so of late. The social relationships and cultural manifestations of nurses as subordinates are there for all to see. Curiously, though, the higher technology areas have seen a more equal partnership between doctors and nurses as doctors have come to trust and value the judgement and knowledge base of nurses based on the close, hour-by-hour, working relationship that is lacking on busy general wards. This equality has tended to be on medicine's terms in many cases, however, as it is technical, biomedical expertise that is valued most by doctors, rather than expertise in caring.

Set against this, the recent moves to reduce junior doctors' hours seem likely to result in a significant range of technical tasks being delegated by doctors to nurses to perform. Many nurses are keen and willing to take on these new tasks – 'the extended role of the nurse', as it used to be known. Is this another example of medical knowledge being the prized currency of practice and the needs of technology (biochemistry tests, venepuncture) driving the subordination of the nurse to the doctor? The nurse will be performing tasks to fulfil the doctor's orders, in other words, nursing subordination to medicine, willingly sought by nurses, exactly as Freire reasoned!

Such subordination is hardly the stuff of which innovative and creative practice will be born as nurses are again following orders.

The much-heralded devolvement of management to ward level has been paralleled in the USA by the development of the nurse entrepreneur. Will this replace some of the caring component of the nursing curriculum in the UK? Devolvement of budgets to ward level means nurses need to know more about budget and resource management, but at the expense of what? Will nursing's slim but growing knowledge base suffer because nurses have to learn more about business studies while delegating care to unregistered health-care assistants? The fragile flower of nursing knowledge can easily be blown aside by management demands that the registered nurse gets on and manages the ward rather than cares for patients. Again the subordinate group loses its identity (nursing) and takes on the content and characteristics of the dominant, as the stuff of management replaces nursing skills. Nursing care in the process becomes devalued and handed down the ladder to the lowest-paid, least-educated. Nursing has indeed participated in its own subordination!

To pick up on the final point in the argument about groups internalizing subordination and making it a need, there is a sense of comfort about knowing that somebody else is taking the responsibility for events. Within the present system it is usually the health authority or trust (i.e. management) or the doctor who is in court if things go wrong. Many nurses are still uncomfortable with the idea of full accountability for their actions and prefer to think of loyalty to the doctors with the medical profession taking the responsibility ultimately. The socialization of women within western society, of course, encourages loyalty as a feminine virtue and encourages the notion that men are the active decision-makers. It is therefore not surprising that there is still a significant undercurrent within nursing that adds up to a need to be subordinate.

It therefore appears that this concept of a subordinate group actively bringing about its own subordination has validity within nursing. As long as this is so, it is hard to see nursing fully developing as an autonomous profession. Rituals will persist and the false messiahs referred to in the first chapter may still be able to introduce new practices, unchallenged and eventually as ritualistic as the practices they claim to replace. Self-awareness as individuals and collectively as a profession of this phenomenon of self-induced subordination, coupled with a strategy for empowerment, does offer a way out of the situation, however.

Obsession with getting the work done and following orders from above without thinking about their meaning too carefully are two instantly recognizable aspects of ritualistic nursing. These behaviours are, according to Freire (1985), characteristic of societies where people are not allowed to take risks and where there is a procedure for everything. Freire was writing about mass society, but could have been writing about nursing when he noted:

Men are lost ... They do not have to think about even the smallest things; there is always some manual that says what to do in situation A or B. Rarely do men have to pause at a street corner to think which direction to follow. There's always an arrow that deproblematizes the situation.

Nursing is trying to escape from precisely that history with qualified nurses taking professional decisions about client care on an individualistic basis, in the light of client needs and the nurse's own knowledge base. Yet there are those in high places who would try and reverse this trend and turn nursing into a mass society, a society where only a few are qualified (registered nurses) and many are not (health-care assistants). If nursing sees a progressive reduction in the number of educated professional nurses and their replacement with an army of willing but inadequately educated assistants, then the mass society of Freire will be upon us. Care will be carried out by people who need detailed manuals for all eventualities, signposts at every street corner and who basically cannot think for themselves. Not only would such care be hopelessly ritualistic and insensitive to individual needs, but it would also be hopelessly inefficient as the professional nurse usually knows what to do immediately without waiting for instructions and orders. Registered nurses are better value for money than health-care assistants!

Transforming nursing practice towards a knowledge-based, client-sensitive and flexible activity requires the nurse to be within the clinical setting and close to the client. This may seem a statement of the obvious but in view of the drive towards nurses becoming business managers and supervisors of assistants (who actually provide the care), it stands repeating. If reclaiming nursing from the bureaucrats involves a revolution, we would dwell upon these words:

Revolution is a critical process, unrealizable without science and reflection. In the midst of reflective action on the world to be transformed, the people come to recognize that the world is indeed being transformed (Freire 1985).

If, by science, we understand the knowledge base of nursing in this context, we are left with the suggestion that a revolution is possible if, whilst carrying out care, nurses think critically about what they are doing, using their own formal knowledge of nursing and their own life experiences. The message is that thinking about what is being done while it is being done makes it possible to see that things can be done differently. Reflection facilitates change. Nurses have the power to revolutionize nursing themselves without waiting for messianic leaders if they will only value the worth of what they do and, of course, question why they do what they do. Praxis in care is possible if nurses can be empowered to collaborate and critically evaluate what nursing is.

Freire has written of vanguardism in his accounts of change and revolution within societies. By this concept he means intellectuals removed from ordinary everyday life setting themselves up as leaders and in the process removing from ordinary people the ability to define their own aims and goals. By laying claim to a monopoly on theoretical leadership, such people merely propagate the divisions they seek to overthrow. It was an understanding of this problem which led Che Guevara, for example, to leave Cuba, disenchanted with Castro and the post-revolutionary state of the island, to seek a new revolution in Bolivia.

Nursing should beware vanguardism for this leads to the false messiahs discussed in our first chapter. If nurses sit back and allow the intellectuals, divorced from clinical reality, to lead nursing, empowerment will not be the result. The hierarchical structure will propagate itself and clinical nurses will not have the power to change the profession. Nurses will still be expected meekly to follow where their betters lead, new ideas will be uncritically implemented, old rituals might persist and new ones will be grafted on to the body of nursing. Those who would *lead* nursing must *do* nursing. Educationalists must engage clinical practice and clinical experts must be valued and acknowledged for all they are worth. Progress along these lines clearly stems from practice and critical reflection upon practice.

Reflection is therefore a key concept in the professional development of nursing for, as de Chardin (1963) stated, it is reflection that turns instinct into thought. Reflection – knowing the self – is the difference between humans and other animals and, as Freire argues, the less reflective a person, the more obstacles he or she will find in the way of liberation. Stereotyped, unthinking nursing care leads to a state of mind that only sees reasons why change is impossible. 'We are too busy, there are not enough staff, the doctors will not like it [has anybody asked them?], we are not covered to do that, we do not do things like that, it is not in the procedure manual' is a familiar litany of excuses obscuring nurses' inability to think and reflect on what they are doing and why.

Reflection upon practice is an essential precursor to nurses collaborating and sharing their knowledge and experience. In this way they may regain control over nursing and so empower nurses to move forwards in creating the new art and science of caring that could be nursing in the next century.

This is therefore an appropriate place to move the argument on from critical social theorists such as Giroux and Freire to the notion of how professionals think in action and how they might usefully reflect upon practice. We will return to critical social theory later to see what further insights it might give into nursing practice, but for now it is the notion of reflection as a means of liberating nursing practice that will form the focus for attention.

If empowerment starts with the recognition that nurses are an oppressed and subordinated group, then the process continues by developing the skills of the reflective practitioner. Nurses need to become knowledgeable doers who can change practice by their own actions and who need to recognize the extent of their knowledge – which may be considerably greater than is given credit in some quarters.

Schon (1983) has argued that many practice-based professions suffer from precisely this lack of recognition due to the dominance of the culture of technical rationality, i.e. the rigorous application of the methods of pure science in a problem-solving approach, within an academic environment. The positivist methods of traditional science are all important and lead to the discovery of knowledge which can be applied by what Glazer (1974) calls the major professions – medicine, engineering, economics and the law. These major professions are grounded in systematic and fundamental science and its accompanying methodology while, in Glazer's view, other professions are regarded as minor in nature because of this lack of scientific grounding.

On this analysis, nursing finds itself in something of a dilemma. It can try and bathe in some of the reflected glory and kudos of the major professions by staying loyally close but subservient to medicine, or it can distance itself from medicine by developing its own knowledge base which incorporates a great deal of qualitative and subjective material like holism and communication skills, but in the process be relegated to the league of minor professions as it lacks a completely scientific foundation.

The major professions depend upon clearly defined outcomes and unambiguous contexts in which they function. Thus, for doctors the outcome is the goal of cure or palliation, within the context usually of a hospital, given the dominant position of hospital-based medicine. Nursing, along with the other minor professions, suffers from ambiguity as there are not usually such clear-cut and simple outcomes to be seen from nursing care. Excellent nursing care is often invisible as it consists of preventing problems from arising. The context within which nursing care occurs is also immensely varied. Nursing does not therefore fit into the major league of professions and consequently frequently finds itself undervalued, ignored and at times patronized. The development of assertive and empowering modes of practice is therefore very difficult on Glazer's analysis of how professions develop and evolve.

Schon (1983) argues that technical rationality breaks down when the outcomes are not clearly defined and the practitioner is not functioning in one simple context, but rather a range of environments. As we have seen, nursing is one such area. Definitions of knowledge that are tied to the rigours of science and laboratory experimental methods are, according to Schon, very narrow and exclude a great deal of knowledge which is derived from practical experience and intuition. Such definitions therefore do professions such as nursing a grave disservice and devalue their true worth. If something is not valued by outsiders then it may come to lack value in the eyes of insiders also and thus we are back to Freire's argument about the subtle ways in which oppressed groups come to participate in their own oppression. To have the confidence to challenge vanguardism in nursing, as well as established rituals, nurses need to value themselves first.

Benner (1984) has argued that nurses know far more than they could ever write down, such is the essence of clinical nursing. This view fits well with Schon's ideas for he argues that we all show in our everyday life knowledge which is not of a rational scientific variety: it is intuitive and spontaneous, demonstrated in our actions. This contrasts with the model of technical rationality which postulates in the first place a body of discrete abstract knowledge which we have to interrogate to find the answer to a problem, and then we apply that knowledge to find a solution in a second stage. While this model can be recognized in action in some areas of nursing, for example in carrying out a pressure sore risk calculation, there are other areas where the nurse's actions are intuitive, almost 'knowledge in action' rather than 'knowledge then action'.

Knowing in action is characterized by spontaneous actions and judgements not involving thinking out in advance: individuals are unaware of a learning process which permits them to act in the observed way and they are unable to describe the knowledge which has been revealed by the action. We are all familiar with the situation where a person is asked 'How did you know to do that?' and can only answer with a shrug of the shoulders. It is suggested that there may be a great deal of invisible nursing knowledge concealed in this way – knowledge which is not even recognized as legitimate knowledge by orthodox medicine because it is not derived from the positivist scientific method.

If this proposition can be validated then there is great empowering potential for nursing contained within this concept. Schon has advanced substantial examples from everyday life to support this concept of knowing in action. Whether it be from the world of art and craft through to sport, excellence is characterized by an absence of formal, scientific knowledge. Whilst not achieving the public acclaim of a Gary Lineker or an Ian Botham, there are many nurses who perform to these levels of excellence, only in a different and more private sphere. They would be just as incapable of telling how they know what they know as Ian Botham would be of explaining some of his momentous achievements on the cricket field or Gary Lineker of explaining how he managed to appear in the right place at the right time to score so many goals. The knowing is in the doing.

Sometimes it is possible consciously to think about what is being done while it is being done: this is known as reflecting in action. Such behaviour is usually associated with an unusual event that makes the practitioner stop and ask 'Why did that happen?' or 'I never noticed that before, what's going on?' The nurse who stops and asks questions such as these becomes a researcher in the practice context. Rather than being bound by the traditional scientific approach of representative sampling and the need to generalize findings across a whole range of situations, the nurse is free to investigate the unique case before him or her. The practitioner builds up expertise on a case-by-case basis as reflection in action becomes central to the art of practice.

The nurse who operates in this way is empowering him- or herself by keeping an open mind, not accepting things at face value, not doing things the way they have always been done, but rather taking each situation on its merits and asking questions of the situation. Why is the person behaving this way? Why have the family suddenly changed their attitudes? What made the client suddenly stop taking the medication? This is reflection in action and can lead to creative, non-ritualistic expert nursing care.

There is therefore a strong case for arguing that nursing knows far more than it is given credit for – the common-sense, intuitive knowing that is inherent in doing rather than formal scientific knowledge, and also the possibility through reflection in action of building up a substantial resource of practice-based knowledge and experience. If these types of knowing can be demonstrated to exist at the same time as the orthodox scientific view of knowledge is challenged, nursing may make significant progress in empowering its practitioners and breaking away from the traditional and ritualistic patterns of action characteristic of a subordinated group.

It is at this stage that the work of Pat Benner (1984) should be examined, for she undertook a major research project which amply demonstrated the existence of the sort of knowledge that Schon has written about. On the first page of her seminal work *From Novice to Expert* (1984), Benner makes the observation that people do not understand the difference between theory and practice in nursing and how nurses learn from practice. She then goes on to weave a rich tapestry of observed nursing practice and show how much of it reveals a great deal of knowledge that is not written down anywhere as formal theory: it is knowledge in action or sometimes intuition. It is also the antithesis of vanguardism.

The key to excellence is that the nurse is allowed to develop and grow individually, building his or her own expertise based on feedback from experience, rather than hidebound by procedure manuals and rules or slavishly following 'experts'. The nurse is free to take reasonable risks and allowed from time to time to fail and even then failure is turned into a positive learning experience as s/he reflects upon why things did not work out. There is almost a positive feedback loop at work here as non-ritualistic practice feeds reflection in action, innovation and creativity, which leads to expertise of the highest order, which in turn leads to non-ritualistic care. Benner's work demonstrates that nursing excellence can exist outside any formal models of knowledge, hence the importance of the art of nursing, or intuition as it may be described.

Consideration of Schon's and Benner's work shows remarkable similarities, although it has to be said that Schon's original book of 374 pages contains only one reference to nursing, noting that it is similar to forestry and meteorology in being a minor profession based directly upon science or containing a high component of science in its educational process. Both authors argue eloquently for another type of knowledge beyond formal scientific knowledge – something that is rooted in and grows out of experience, and which is neither valued nor recognized by traditional orthodoxy as represented, for example, by medical science.

The recognition by nursing first of all, and then by others, of this valuable and rich resource may substantially help to empower nurses and underline the importance of practice-based knowledge that is both flexible and creative. Such knowledge will also allow nurses to reclaim nursing for itself and encourage the generation of nursing from within the body of nursing, rather than from charismatic leaders who fall victim to the trap of vanguardism.

After reading the preceding section, it might be reasonable to ask if practice-based knowledge is so important, what is the need for formal education? Why not place nurses in the wards and community and let them learn from experience as apprentices in the traditional way?

The key to rejecting this simple suggestion is to understand the nature of the ward experience. Gadamer (1970) defined experience as the turning around of preconceptions that are not met by actual situations. There is first an element of activity in this definition: the student is an active participant in thinking about and making sense of the situation, the student is called upon to reflect both on and in action. This is very different from the traditional perceptions of student experience, which is about getting on with the work and not asking questions. In the traditional sense, the student is not encouraged to engage the clinical situation in meaningful dialogue, asking why things happen the way they do and how they might be done differently. Students simply follow orders and do what they are told.

The second key element is the notion of preconceptions – the student comes to the situation with some prior knowledge or ideas and tests them out in practice. This prior knowledge has to be acquired somewhere, such as a classroom under the guidance of a teacher who can ensure it is relevant to the situations to be encountered. Students can also explore with the teacher the meanings of the experience after the placement, raising their self-awareness in the process. Experience is therefore educationally meaningful for students when they come to a placement prepared with some knowledge which they can then test out in practice, reflecting upon and questioning that practice, with the help of the clinical staff and their teacher.

Benner proposes that nurses grow into expert practitioners from novices over many years and through a series of well-defined phases. Thus the student beginning as an absolute novice learns to follow rules exactly and is therefore limited and inflexible in practice. As the nurse recognizes patterns of behaviour that recur in patients and begins to attach meanings associated with this patterning, s/he may be said to move towards advanced beginner status where, for example, guidelines can begin to be applied as the student builds up enough experience to make sense of them. Rules, though, still need to be closely observed and the student can only focus on one aspect of a situation at a time. As the nurse reaches the stage of being able to plan logically and analytically for patient care, prioritizing problems and looking ahead, the stage of competence has been reached and when the nurse is able to grasp whole situations in one, rather than considering its constituent parts one by one, the stage of proficiency is arrived at. Finally, the expert nurse, in Benner's terminology, is able to function apparently without rules; she or he just seems to know what to do automatically. The knowing is in the doing, as Schon would say.

The road to expertise mapped out by Benner is heavily dependent upon practical knowledge acquired in the clinical situation. However, it had to start with some formal, abstract knowledge: the student needed guidance and support from clinical staff and teachers, ideas had to be checked and validated, the self had to be explored. In short, there was a need for a formal educational foundation and continuing support along the way. Expertise is not gained by clinical practice alone; there has to be an alliance with formal theory that recognizes the value of experience.

In reviewing the preceding pages it should be possible to see that there are powerful linkages between writers from very different backgrounds initially but who focus together on empowerment within nursing. Freire makes us aware that nurses are an oppressed group and points out some of the ways in which we are oppressed without even realizing it, pointing to the need for education and reflection upon action as a means of liberation. Schon strongly argues precisely this case for reflection upon action, demonstrating that professions such as nursing are undervalued because the nature of much of our knowledge falls outside the conventional orthodoxy of science, being founded in practice and reflection upon that practice. Benner brings nursing sharply into focus by describing the ways in which nurses know far more than they can ever write down about nursing, showing that expert nursing is derived from the interaction between formal education, practice and reflection upon that practice. Expert nursing, as we have noted, also suffers from the disadvantage of being invisible as it usually acts to prevent problems arising.

Education can help nursing realize its liberty, and carried out as an integral part of practice, help nursing shed its ritualistic trappings whilst ensuring that the future does not see us taking on a new collection of rituals as we get rid of the old. The key is empowerment, to feel that as nurses we can question and challenge conventional science-based wisdom and also assert our own professional self-confidence in the future by questioning new ideas and concepts as they appear on the health-care scene. Empowerment is about rejecting the traditional view of power which leads only to oppression and subordination which, as we have seen, in their turn lead to ritualistic, routinized behaviour and the silencing of the subordinated group as they lose their voices and critical faculties. Approaching nursing from a perspective that recognizes our subordination and its effects is the first step to redressing the balance. Following on from this self-awareness and insight into nursing's situation, collaboration between practice and education may help raise our own self-esteem and allow nursing to liberate itself from the last century of domination by outside forces.

In this chapter we have considered a range of issues around empowerment from a critical social perspective and seen that the notion of nurses having more knowledge than they can ever say, if explicated fully, is vital to our future. It could act as a counterbalance against those who would lead nursing into paths that denigrate caring when compared to biomedicine on the one hand and those who, despite losing touch with clinical reality, still think they know nursing enough to act as leaders. This latter group of intellectuals could mislead nursing and lead to nurses trading one set of rituals for another. It is time for a change within nursing – it is time to empower the clinical nurse.

References

Benner P (1984) *From Novice to Expert*. New York, Addison Wesley.
de Chardin P (1963) *El Fenomeno humano*. Madrid, Taurus.
Freire P (1970) *The Pedagogy of the Oppressed*. New York, Seabury Press.
Freire P (1985) *The Politics of Education; Culture, Power and Liberation* (translated by Macedo). New York, Macmillan.
Gadamer G (1970) *Truth and Method*. London, Sheer and Ward.
Glazer N (1974) *Schools of the Minor Professions*. New York, Minerva.
Giroux A (1985) Introduction. In: Freire P (ed) *The Politics of Education*. New York, Macmillan.
Schon D (1983) *The Reflective Practitioner*. New York, Basic Books.

4 *Nursing and change*

Introduction

In the opening chapter we alluded to an interesting paradox concerning nursing. It has a reputation for being a very traditional and reactionary profession, yet it also appears to be capable of suddenly embracing some new ideas, leading to radical change with little or no consideration of whether the change it has embarked upon has any evidence to support it. This latter characteristic is also shared by the Department of Health as government ministers reform management structures in one fell swoop one year (Griffiths) before changing everything again almost the next (NHS reforms 1991). Why is nursing therefore so resistant to change and apparently able to make huge changes simultaneously? This Janus-faced paradox will be explored in this chapter, which will look at theories of change and how relevant they are to nursing in practice. A possible answer will be provided later.

The need for a critical evaluation of ideas about change is important if nurses are to be able to plot a course between the two extremes of 'all change, like it or not' and an 'over my dead body, always done it this way' attitude to change. Perhaps the authoritarian, hierarchical nature of the NHS helps to explain the apparent rapidity with which management-imposed change occurs while the enthusiasm and bright ideas of clinical staff are frequently dashed to pieces by the apathy or discouraging attitudes of others. Change, when it appears to occur, is driven by those with least knowledge about direct client care and NHS management, yet those with most knowledge about care – clinicians – can find their ideas blocked by their clinical peers and colleagues. Perhaps a consideration of theories about change will shed some light on the matter. This is essential as otherwise attempts at empowerment will lead only to frustration and demotivation while an underworld of ritualistic practice continues despite superficial change that owes more to political expediency, coercion, charismatic individuals and cosmetics than it does to reality.

Change in nursing can occur at several different levels, the most important of which is the one-to-one, nurse-to-patient level. Ultimately this is what nursing comes down to – the way a nurse communicates with and cares for a patient and his or her family. Practice on this level may be changed by the introduction of a health education package or a new type of dressing, for example. On a slightly larger scale, the next level of change affects groups of nurses such as ward and community teams and how they organize their care. Issues here are more about who delivers care and how this is organized rather than the nature of that care, although clearly the who and the how exert strong influences over what that care consists of. Changes in skill mix or introducing primary nursing are possible examples. Change then works on collections of nursing teams at the level of the hospital or trust, such as moving to clinical directorates or patient-focused hospital initiatives. Finally, nursing is subject to change in the national picture, both formally under the Department of Health such as introducing Project 2000 and less formally, such as responding to changes in junior doctors' hours.

It is easy in these latter three cases to forget about the nature of nursing and concentrate instead on attempting to change social systems and organizations, especially as much change theory is written from this perspective as part of management studies.

At all levels, therefore, nurses may find themselves as the originators of change or as the subjects of change responding to the initiatives of others. Too often nurses have been the latter rather than the former. The effects of change may just be confined to the nurse and patient or they may spread throughout a wide circle of people with increasingly unpredictable consequences. This latter observation stems from the field of chaos theory: a small change in one part of a system may have massive and totally unpredictable consequences elsewhere (Gleick, 1987). This is known as sensitive dependence upon initial conditions and is well-illustrated by the traditional rhyme cited as long ago as 1758 by Benjamin Franklin:

For want of a nail the shoe was lost,
For want of a shoe the horse was lost,
For want of a horse the rider was lost,
For want of a rider the battle was lost,
For want of a battle the kingdom was lost.

Shakespeare cites the best-known example of losing a horse in battle, as Richard III bewails his fate at Bosworth Field! The world is not the mechanistic and predictable place positivist science once thought and the nurse, upon reflection, might be able to think of a range of examples in nursing which echo these erstwhile words of Richard III. The unpredictability and uncertainty which are generated by change are, as we shall see, key agents in producing opposition to change.

Changing cultures

Any account on the subject of change usually addresses this essential topic as either the culture itself is the direct target of a change strategy or it is recognized that to make more concrete, although perhaps smaller changes, this less tangible entity of culture also has to change. One simple definition of culture is that it consists of the commonly held beliefs, attitudes and values that exist within an organization (Williams *et al.* 1989).

It will be recalled that we have already suggested that one of the reasons why nursing has found it hard to change is that much of what was taken as nursing knowledge in the past was actually only nurses' attitudes and beliefs. Traditional knowledge about nursing may therefore be viewed, in light of these authors, as more of a culture of nursing. It is salutary therefore to note that Williams *et al.* go on to note that the culture of an organization is self-sealing, an embedded product of past strategy which acts to negate any future strategy requiring change. The rites, rituals and symbols of an organization are all manifestations of that culture which pervades all aspects of decision-making and practice.

Hierarchical respect for, and deference to, authority are immediately seen as characteristics of nursing culture. The symbols of nursing uniform which are Victorian and originate in domestic service express a very outmoded and traditional sort of culture. The rites and rituals of nursing were explored by the current authors elsewhere (Walsh and Ford, 1989) and the picture that emerges is one of nurses as a group whose culture dictates that they follow orders. There are many situations when not to do so would be dangerous of course, but there are many other situations when orders as such are totally inappropriate and serve only to highlight the hierarchical nature of power relationships within this culture. There are other situations in which orders should be questioned and perhaps a request, rather than an order, might have been more appropriate in the first place.

Changing a culture such as this is essential if any real changes in practice are to follow, and clearly change is going to be difficult. Williams *et al.* offer the following list of key characteristics possessed by cultures: it is important to understand these factors before attempting to devise strategies for change.

Culture is first influenced by the environment both within and without the group or organization. Internal environment is concerned with recruitment and training of staff in colleges of nursing, behaviours of other staff in clinical areas and the decision-making and control systems within nursing, while the external environment considers the context within which nursing has to function. Government policy towards the NHS and nurse staffing levels, legal constraints and the medical profession's perceptions of nurses are examples of these external factors. The socialization process that affects nurses as students is familar to us all as students 'learn the ropes' and discover the hidden agenda that enables them to survive, sadly often at the expense of their ideals, in the clinical area. This hidden agenda may involve the student keeping his/her head down and mouth shut if a satisfactory report is required – hardly conducive to change.

Culture also has both input and output components in that it is the product of certain attitudes and beliefs about nursing (input) which in turn leads to certain actions (output). This output then feeds back into the original attitudes and belief systems (see p. 18). These characteristics make nursing very resistant to change as they tend to lead to self-fulfilling prophecies. For example, 'We treat pressure sores this way because we believe it is the right way and this is the way we have always done it, so why do things any differently?' Williams *et al.* note that career-based organizations with standardized selection procedures and training programmes operating in a relatively stable market with low staff turnover are most likely to be change-resistant as a result of this input–output cycle. These characteristics are recognizable in varying degrees in nursing, especially in those areas most resistant to change.

History is a major determinant of culture and nursing bears elegant testimony to this assertion as the effects of its origins in religious houses and the military can still be seen today in its obsession with hierarchy. There is a partly unconscious element about culture; basic assumptions become assimilated to the point that we are unaware they exist. Thus, for example, the ward sister still frequently accompanies the consultant on the ward round. It is just assumed to be natural, but often there are more important nursing activities that require the sister's time. If primary or team nursing is in place the primary nurse or team leader could join the round for his or her patients only or alternatively attend a case conference or review meeting, allowing the doctors to conduct a purely medical round. This would represent a better use of nursing time and ensure that any nursing input to the ward round or case conference came from the nurse who knew most about the patient.

Not all the beliefs, attitudes and values that make up a culture may be commonly held by all individuals as some may be peculiar to differing subgroups of the overall organization. Intensive care or theatres may have differences compared to a care of the elderly unit while students may have differences in culture compared to sisters and charge nurses. The culture of nursing is therefore not likely to be homogeneous; there will be significant differences between specialisms, units, grades of staff and parts of the country. Any approach to change must recognize this variety.

This discussion of nursing suggests that it fits well into mainstream models of organizational culture and does so in such a way that it has most of the characteristics of a culture that is going to be extremely resistant to change. The next step is therefore to explore some of the strategies for change that have been proposed and see how applicable they might be to nursing.

Approaches to change

Rational decision-making: a linear model

Our first port of call will be the rational decision-making organizational model that management typically uses in response to a major crisis or problem. Management in this model initially start with a mission statement which highlights the type of organization they see themselves as and the fundamental purpose which underpins the very existence of the organization. The issues are then addressed in an assessment and problem diagnosis exercise. This leads to formulation of possible solutions and choices being made between the alternatives. The next stage, having selected a choice, is to plan its implementation before proceeding to effect the necessary interventions and finally evaluate their effectiveness in achieving the desired changes.

This model is sometimes referred to as a linear approach as things move in a straight line from one stage to the next. Reality is very different as life is rarely so simple. This model has been criticized for its oversimplification and in practice there is a great deal of movement back and forth between stages as they are all interdependent. Further, the circumstances are usually changing all the time as management work on the problems. Often the very presence of management distorts the picture or they see an untypical situation or do not understand what they are seeing. These sort of criticisms are levelled at some management teams engaged in skill mix reprofiling exercises, for example.

If one stage of this process goes wrong, then it is likely that all subsequent stages go wrong as they are interdependent in a chain-reaction manner. The system is in danger of becoming mechanistic and inflexible. Errors made in the assessment and diagnosis stage can therefore lead to disastrous results in the implementation stage. Sensitive dependence upon initial conditions may magnify a small error at one stage into a huge mistake later on. A further difficulty is that, if management are seen to be leading the movement for change, especially if they adopt an authoritarian approach in considering choices, staff may be resentful or indifferent, resulting in poor outcomes after change implementation.

This rational, logical problem-solving approach to change suffers from other difficulties also, for as Sheehan (1990) points out, it contains the inherent assumption that people are rational and logical also. We know they are not, however. People, including nurses, continue to eat too much and not take enough exercise; they smoke and drink and drive their cars too fast. In short, they are logical and rational only some of the time, not all of the time. Logic and rationality are described by Sheehan as necessary for change but not sufficient in themselves, whatever model of change is being used. Human irrationality cannot be ignored in planning strategies for change.

The preceding discussion should have sounded very familiar for this account also fits the nursing process. What is care if it is not a change process? The aim of nursing care, whichever theoretical model of nursing is considered, is to change the client's health status for the better. In that sense all nursing care is about change and the nursing process is derived from this linear, organizational change and problem-solving model with the nurse as 'management' and the patient as 'staff'. The implications of this for nursing care are that if this change model is criticized as flawed in terms of organizational change, might the same criticisms also apply to the nursing process? Are there other models of organizational change which by analogy could be applied to nursing to produce different patterns and approaches to care? This issue will be explored further in Chapter 9.

Lewin's force field theory of change

There is however a second way of thinking about change and that stems from the ideas of Kurt Lewin (1951). He suggested thinking of change as the product of two sets of opposing forces, one driving change and the other resisting change. This model is therefore different from the linear model as a range of factors and influences are all acting at once and any change that occurs depends upon the sum of all these forces. No change occurs when these forces are in equilibrium but change will occur if the forces resisting it are weakened or the forces driving it are strengthened, or both. This notion is referred to as a force field theory of change as it sees change occurring only when the normal balance of forces is disturbed in favour of change.

Lewin also offers a three-stage model for disturbing this equilibrium in such a way that change is possible. Stage 1 consists of unfreezing the status quo and this involves making the case for change by showing the inadequacies of the present system. In the example given in Figure 4.1, staff have to demonstrate the shortcomings of whatever system is used for care delivery. Do mix-ups happen because staff leave things to each other while nobody is actually taking responsibility for a patient or conversely is there confusion due to duplication of effort? Is there evidence of deterioration in standards as measured by complaints, pressure sores, patient falls, etc.? Are sickness rates unacceptably high? Are student evaluations very critical?

The next stage is to act on the two sets of forces, weakening those resisting change and strengthening those that support change. This latter goal might involve organizing a ward seminar, sending another member of staff to a study day, distributing literature on the ward and encouraging students to share with staff what they have learnt in college about primary nursing. Simultaneously, enrolled nurses might be brought into the process and their position discussed: if they can be made to feel valued members of the team with a major role to play, this might reduce their resistance.

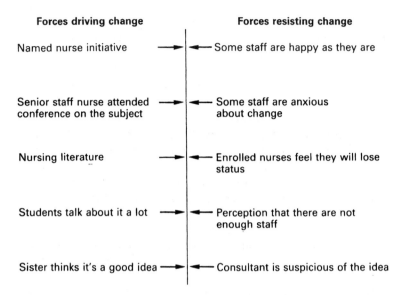

Figure 4.1 *Lewin's force field theory of change. In this example, the forces involved for a ward considering introducing primary nursing are shown*

Consultation, discussion and information-sharing could help reduce uncertainty and anxiety; paper exercises might address the staffing issue to show that the off-duty can be made to work realistically, whilst a discussion with the consultant might allay fears that perhaps nurses were about to usurp medical authority. In ways such as this the balance of forces can be tilted so as to favour change.

The third and final stage involves making sure that the changes made stick; in other words, refreezing the situation. This requires that the forces changed are the ones that will remain changed. There is therefore little point in bringing in, say, a primary nurse coordinator from outside to set up the system for as soon as that person leaves the ward, things will slide backwards. Consequently all the regular staff must be taken along by the change; literature should continue to be available as it is published; when another study day is advertised, another member of staff should go; student involvement while on placement should be a regular feature. The forces to concentrate upon are those that will continue to be present after the change process is over as these must be refrozen in the new configuration if the change is to persist.

Within the context of identifying resistant forces it is worth noting that Williams *et al.* (1989) suggest that key factors are people not realizing the need for change, anxiety and uncertainty produced by change and a failure to take into account how people behave within organizational settings. With regard to this latter point, Kotter and Schlesinger (1986) have proposed that people may fear a personal loss within the organization and feel change is not needed or does not make any sense and that they lack the ability to adapt to change.

In Chapter 1 we explored a list of reasons which tend to make people unaware of the need for change, such as traditional nurse training rather than education and all the historical reasons which predispose many nurses to follow orders rather than look for different, new ways of doing things. If nurses operated as reflective practitioners (Chapter 3), looking at what they were doing and thinking about their practice, it might be easier for them to see the need for change. Chapter 3 also looked at critical social theory, which suggests that a characteristic of subordinated groups such as nursing is to take on a watered-down version of the characteristics of the dominant group (medicine) and to be unable to realize they are subordinated, thereby reducing the realization of the need for change. Familiarization with the ideas espoused by critical theory would predispose staff to be looking for change as part of their everyday job.

One other factor which, if absent, also reduces the realization that change is needed is the setting of standards. If a ward does not have standards, how can staff realize they are failing to achieve and therefore that their practice is in need of change? Setting standards is a topic to be explored in Chapter 6, but it is suggested now that this is a very powerful method of driving change by bringing home to people the need for change.

The issue of staff uncertainty may be tackled by giving information and discussing ideas fully with staff so that they can explore where the changes might lead and how they as individuals might be affected. It is a very strong argument for bottom-up, rather than top-down, change – a topic that will be explored shortly. In this way nurses become empowered as power is shared and each nurse begins to feel that s/he matters and has a say in the change. Another key factor in reducing staff uncertainty is that those seen as leading change must have credibility in the eyes of staff affected. General managers have no credibility when it comes to changing nursing practice in any way as they are not nurses, but there again, how much clinical credibility do some nurse managers or educationalists have? Staff need to feel the change agent knows what he or she is talking about if they are to have confidence and trust in what is being proposed. The development of clinical practice through initiatives such as the English Nursing Board Higher Award and nurse practitioners should facilitate change by increasing the number of nurses with the credibility to lead change in clinical practice.

Consideration of organizations suggests that, while it is essential to change the attitudes and beliefs of key people in authority such as managers, change must also be owned by the staff, who should feel they have a stake in it. This is what is meant by bottom-up change rather than top-down, management-led change. The original (disastrous) implementation of the nursing process in the late 1970s was a classic example of top-down change. To overcome resistance, the areas of bottom-up change management and attitude change now need to be addressed.

Bottom-up change

The bottom-up view of changing nursing practice is consistent with the empowering, sharing approach outlined earlier and very different from the traditional top-down style. The bottom-up approach has been advocated in nursing by Driscoll (1982), who called it a normative–re-educative style of change, the key characteristic of which is pressure from within groups to alter practice. Teaching and learning are by implication important dimensions of the change process as the group of staff grow and own the change.

A well-written critique of the traditional, management-led approach to change has been provided by Lupton (1986), who argues that however much managers say they will consult widely, talk to staff and listen to their views, in the end it is always managers who make the decisions, excluding other staff in the process. This hierarchical view of change based upon management prerogative is still widespread and leads management into the position of having to make changes while preserving their prerogative, and at the same time keeping staff who have no control over the change interested in the process and outcomes of change. It will be seen that this is a tall order.

This top-down view is not capable of seeing things from the staff's perspective. If it was, it might see that in addition to the formal structures of management, there is also a lot of informal manage-ment, of staff by staff, taking place. Sister may be in her office, but the auxiliaries and students work their own ways out of organizing time and work, often without Sister being aware. There is often an alternative management structure, a pecking order built upon who has been there longest and force of personality, rather than qualifications, grades and job descriptions. Failure to explore this alternative management structure can lead to the failure of any change project as key areas of resistance may go unobserved, while possible positive forces for change might also go unnoticed.

Lupton considers this concept of top-down management prerogative is inappropriate in the modern world, arrogant and distasteful. In his view it is a major obstacle to change as it does not necessarily confer upon managers wisdom that is greater than non-managers may possess. Tennyson in *Locksley Hall* observed that 'knowledge comes but wisdom lingers'; in other words, knowledge may be forgotten, but wisdom is not. Knowledge of management may be learnt and is therefore in that sense part of a management prerogative, but wisdom is different and is accessible without formal training in management. All nurses have wisdom and if progress is to be made towards changing nursing in such a way that it is flexible and adaptable enough to keep pace with the changes in health-care need, this process can only begin from the location where nursing takes place in everyday practice, the nurse–patient interaction. The value to the cause of change of the reflective practitioner, working in an empowered way, is therefore enormous.

The bottom-up view of change emphasizes the involvement of staff with real shared power to make decisions. The aim should be to discover what is happening now and why, before addressing the issue of change. Efforts should be directed towards team building and cooperation as this will maximize flexibility and minimize conflict whilst permitting individuals, within a supportive team environment, to give of their best. This approach will also be recognized as consistent with the feminist approaches discussed in Chapter 2 and, given the team nature of many nursing environments, has much therefore to commend it as an approach to change.

Flexibility is a recurring theme in this discussion about the advantages of a bottom-up approach to change and this is emphasized by Peters and Waterman (1986), who argue that successful organizations build fluidity into their structures in order to acquire a bias for action. They are critical of bureaucratic methods with a succession of formal committees and reports that stifle the life out of an idea. They argue for an 'adhocracy' concerned with getting on with the job and getting results in which there is open, rapid and intense communication and a loose, fluid structure which leads to a bias for action rather than a formal bureaucracy, focusing on report-writing and committees.

These authors encourage change by the process of 'chunking', a style commonplace in Japanese industry which relies for its success upon small flexible sections who are given enough autonomy to get on and solve their own problems. Change occurs incrementally as smaller problems are solved by blitzing them with intensive effort, involving anybody who might have a contribution to make regardless of rank and status. Once staff see that small problems can be solved and that change is possible, this fosters a 'can do' attitude and staff will be prepared to tackle slightly larger problems. Nurses should be familiar with this concept in care-planning where difficult-to-achieve, long-term patient goals are broken down into easier, smaller, short-term goals. Ward and community teams make ideal sections in the Japanese sense and, given the autonomy, could well make substantial inroads into larger problems affecting whole hospitals or trusts, such as reducing pressure sore incidence and readmission rates.

Peters and Waterman argue that successful change comes from trying things out rather than in-depth analysis, talks, seminars, reports, working groups and committees. Experimentation is a cheap form of learning in their view. This means that there has to be permission to fail and within health care there are obvious ethical limitations to experimentation which might not apply in industry. However, there are strong arguments that economies of scale and bureaucratic empire-building inhibit change, whilst breaking things down into flexible smaller pieces and encouraging staff to work out their own solutions promote successful change. Such a style is also consistent with the principles of empowerment explored earlier and will have a greater probability of success if staff are used to working in a reflective mode. Staff who regularly think about what they are doing, take time to step back and ask why and how are more likely to be able to achieve successful change within this flexible action-oriented framework.

Attitude change

To have any value, theories of change must also recognize the humanity of the subjects of change – people. As such there are a

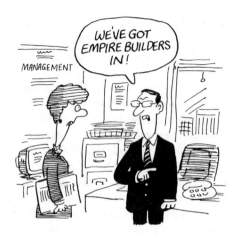

range of complex psychological and social forces at work which can defeat the most carefully laid strategy and implemented plans. It is the area of attitudes and beliefs that often holds the key to the success of change.

Changing attitudes is at the crux of any plan to change nursing, for in addition to the various views of change theory under discussion in this chapter, nursing itself frequently confuses attitudes and associated beliefs with knowledge. Nursing action is often the result therefore of attitudes and beliefs rather than knowledge. This is not to decry the role of intuition within nursing practice, which authors such as Benner (1984) have pointed out is essential.

If change is attempted by explaining the need for change and justifying each step logically, seeking to measure outcomes, this is known as the rational–empirical model and unfortunately, as we have seen, it often fails because humans are not rational. The top-down management-directed power-coercion style rarely fares any better in reality as, while staff may appear to change in order to keep the boss happy, in practice they often carry on as before with change occurring only at a superficial level. One of the principal causes that lies behind the failure of these two approaches is the difficulty of changing attitudes. The bottom-up, normative–re-educative approach involving staff has the advantage of being susceptible to attitude change, however.

Cognitive dissonance theory (see p. 20) suggests attitudes may be changed if a situation can be created in which a person acts in such a way as to be inconsistent with what he or she thinks.

Dissonance is defined as an adverse emotional state by Stroebe and Jonas (1988). It refers to a way of thinking (cognition) that runs counter to the required action. For example, a student who is strongly opposed to euthanasia may be asked in a classroom debate to argue the case in favour. This student is carrying out an act that s/he thinks is wrong, and will probably feel unhappy and uncomfortable about the prospect; there is therefore a state of dissonance. The opposite of dissonance is consonance and this involves thoughts that are consistent with actions.

The student in the example above may act to try and increase consonance by, for example, thinking that putting up a good argument will avoid disapproval from tutorial staff and will help towards writing a forthcoming essay which will be on this topic. This will enable the student to argue the case for euthanasia based on consonance. However, if there is no essay on the topic to be written and the lecturer has given the impression that there are no negative connotations involved in refusing to take part, the student will experience dissonance. Psychologists also predict that the less the benefit from taking part, the greater will be the dissonance as it is harder for the person to justify behaving in a way that is against his or her thinking and attitudes.

Psychological theory, which is well-supported by experimental evidence, predicts that people try and reduce dissonance because it is an unpleasant experience. If individuals are unable to alter their patterns of action, then they have to change their way of thinking about the actions they are involved in; in other words, their attitudes towards the relevant actions. Dissonance therefore leads to attitude change.

A great deal of psychological research has gone into the effects of dissonance and attitude change. Stroebe and Jonas (1988) have summarized this complex but crucial experimental area as follows. The magnitude of attitude change in people who are induced to behave in a way which is against their attitudes is increased if:

1. Incentives in performing the task were high but the person had little choice about performing the task.
2. Incentives in performing the task were low but the person had a large degree of freedom of choice about performance.

In situation 1, dissonance is low but there is a high degree of consonance and the reward acts to induce attitude change, whilst in situation 2 dissonance is high and it is this which induces attitude change.

The implications for nursing are that to pursue the goal of attitude change amongst nurses it is necessary to induce a change of practice under conditions in which the individual is not *forced* to comply. The dissonance thus set up will most likely be resolved by the individual having to bring his or her attitude into line with practice. The alternative approach involves giving the nurse little or no choice in the matter but relying on large incentives to induce attitude change.

The type 2 approach is more in line with the empowering philosophy that underpins this book, although the authors acknowledge the validity of the type 1 method (p. 71). Inducing change in practice, in a situation in which it is not compulsory, is uncommon in the traditional nursing world of hierarchies and orders. Sadly, this is the most effective way of changing attitude through dissonance.

The reader might want to pause and reflect upon some major nursing changes that have been made and analyse them within this framework. For example, the implementation of the nursing process was carried out under conditions of no choice but with no perceived rewards or benefits for staff. Not surprisingly, therefore, the attitude of many nurses has remained hostile to this concept. The 'no choice, no reward' case is unfortunately often the way of things in nursing; hence the difficulty in changing attitudes.

The need to persuade staff to change practice, even if only for an experimental period, while retaining the freedom to opt out, suggests that education will be a most powerful tool in this approach to change. This is consistent with the normative–re-educative approach discussed earlier. Exploring the need for change in a supportive group environment which is free from hierarchies and where the members feel valued and important could achieve a great deal. This is, of course, very different from traditional nurse training. If members of a nursing team operating in this empowering way value their experiences in nursing and reflect upon them in reviewing practice, this too will facilitate a willingness to try something new, as will a flexible 'bias for action' ward culture (Peters and Waterman, 1986). Hierarchies and power-conscious individuals will only interfere with this educative process which can prepare the way for a change in practice which in turn can lead to a change in attitude.

There are striking parallels between this approach and the force field theory discussed earlier of Lewin. Attitude change can reduce forces opposing change and enhance forces in favour. The unfreezing process corresponds to this educational–discussion stage which sets up the change while the refreezing process after the change corresponds to the new attitudes which may be created. Attitudes tend to be stable and lasting – another key ingredient in Lewin's views of change which emphasizes the need for freezing into the new situation components which will last, if the change is to persist.

In emphasizing the positive role that education can play in setting the scene for attitude change it is necessary to insert a note of caution, for as Freire (1985) has argued, education can also be used as a means of social control dedicated to preserving the status quo. The discussion in Chapter 3 of Freire's ideas on education should be borne in mind together with the well-known maxim of Marx that the educators should also be educated. Freire argues strongly that the world is not a given place but is constantly changing and in the making, hence the importance of people participating critically in transforming actions, or conscientization.

From a nursing perspective these ideas advocate the involvement of all in the process of change, but also suggest to nurses that they should read and listen to information they are being given as part of the change process with a healthy scepticism, particularly if the source of the information is management. They may be pursuing their own political agenda and therefore be placing a particular slant on information or perhaps be less than educated themselves in the matters they talk about. Material that arises from within the nursing team such as experiential learning based upon reflection on practice is more likely to fuel meaningful change that benefits nursing practice and patient care. If outside people are brought in to talk about new ideas, nurses should check their credentials: are they qualified to talk as experts? Information derived from the nursing journals should also be checked for credibility. Not all research is sound research!

If nurses take these cautionary words to heart, it can be seen that the road to changing attitudes starts with collaboration amongst the nursing team using discussion and education as a means of establishing the need for change, without any element of compulsion. Changing practice in this way, even if only for an experimental period, may well produce significant shifts in attitude which may then lead to the new approaches becoming seen as normal and supported by positive staff attitudes.

One final piece of the jigsaw is provided from the field of action research. This approach to research involves the subjects of research – in this case nurses – as active participants in the research process. The researcher acts as a facilitator working alongside staff, talking with them and exploring their feelings as the investigation proceeds. This is similar to participant observation styles of research but there is a key difference in that no attempt is made to conceal the role of the researcher and participants become actively involved in the study. A wide range of methods can be used, drawing upon either the empirical tradition (e.g. staff questionnaires) or the qualitative approach (e.g. in-depth patient interviews). It is this sense of collaboration and active participation that makes action research different from other methodologies and entirely consistent with the bottom-up approach to change that has been proposed so far in this chapter.

This style of research in nursing has been advocated by several authors such as Webb (1989) who argued that it permitted nurses to tackle problems in the clinical area themselves, working towards changes and practical solutions which are then owned by the staff. The added bonus is that it permits staff to learn about the research process on the way. For Webb, action research is potentially a very fruitful method of introducing change to nursing. Towell and Harries (1979) have also stressed the sense of empowerment that comes from nurses solving their own problems and clarifying their own roles in this way rather than relying on outside 'experts'. The reader is reminded of earlier observations about following false prophets.

Action research on its own will not change practice, however. An example of a study which in the end failed was that of Hunt (1987) who used nurse teachers to try and change mouth care and preoperative fasting routines by locating research articles and then working through formal education and the Procedures and Supplies Committees.

Ward staff refused to change as they felt more secure with established routines. The adverse effects of stress and anxiety tending to block change must be acknowledged here. There are, however, several other contributory reasons that might explain this failure. If the ward staff saw the tutors and formal education as authority, then the power-coercion model of change is at work which, as we know, is not usually successful except at a superficial level. If staff felt they had no choice about change, but saw little reward in making the change, dissonance theory suggests there would have been little change in attitude, therefore little long-term change in practice. The presence of formal committee structures suggests the sort of bureaucratic obstacles that Peters and Waterman predict will block change. Given these factors and the lack of home-grown, ward-based ownership of change, nurse tutors going into a ward advocating change is a top-down model. It is therefore not surprising that this worthy effort at change failed.

The chapter so far has argued strongly for change to be seen as something that is most likely to succeed if it is a participative venture involving all staff. The requirement to establish the need for change is recognized as crucial along with the involvement of staff on a voluntary basis. This is most likely to lead to the sort of attitude changes that are essential to underpin change. This bottom-up approach is consistent with the principles of empowerment, reflective practice and liberation nursing based upon critical awareness that have been explored so far. Coercive models of change often make only superficial differences and propagate the established top-down power structures that block true change and the development of the nursing profession, while rational–empirical models suffer from the problem that human beings are not always rational.

To conclude this chapter, it is worth looking at some recent case studies of change in the literature to see how the ideas discussed so far relate to real, researched nursing situations.

Examples of change

Change is nowhere more apparent than in the field of nursing education, therefore it is instructive to examine the research of Davis (1991) who looked at the effects of the changes brought about by the merger of two schools of nursing to make a new college. Davis was concerned by how individuals saw change as he was particularly struck by an observation made by Marris (1975) that individuals facing change will tend to have an immediate reaction of opposition and an impulse of rejection that must be allowed to play itself out before meaningful change can occur. Marris points out that rational explanations are not enough in themselves to overcome initial resistance which then leads to individuals in authority resorting to a coercive approach to change and all the weaknesses that are inherent in that method.

Davis therefore considers that change will mean different things to different people and may even mean different things to the same person at different times, leading to a perception of ambivalence. This was indeed one of his main findings amongst the mixture of students, tutors and support staff he interviewed by questionnaire (totalling 67 out of a possible 78 subjects, a very good response rate). Other key factors to emerge were a recognition that, with the advent of Project 2000, change was necessary but that there was a lack of information, consultation and grass-roots involvement, whilst some individuals were using the change process for personal gain by empire-building. The change taking place was seen as top-down and operating within a hierarchical structure whilst it was taking place too quickly and with insufficient planning. Factors such as stress and poor communication were also identified.

These perceptions will not be unfamiliar to many nurse educators and, as Davis points out, it is not so much the reality of change that matters as the staff's perception of the situation. As long as staff *perceive* change as being top-down and management-driven with little regard for consultation, that is sufficient to antagonize staff towards the changes proposed, even if in management's view this is not the case. A second important observation by Davis was that staff broadly fell into two categories – those who were active and those who were passive with regard to the change process. This is a simplification of the concept expressed by Rogers and Shoemaker (1971) who felt that people's responsiveness to change could be expressed along a continuum from innovators and early adapters at one end through the majority who eventually fall into line at varying speeds to the laggards, sceptics and finally those who reject and actively oppose change at the other extreme.

The picture painted by Davis is a familiar NHS one of top-down change which has failed consequently to involve staff with any sense of ownership. There was little opportunity to choose whether or not to participate in the change, which suggests that, according to dissonance theory, unless large rewards are forthcoming, there will be little change in attitude, the vital ingredient for successul change. This hierarchical approach led Davis to suggest that future amalgamations and other major changes in education should involve a management style based upon expertise in managing change rather than reliant upon hierarchy. He argues strongly for the facilitation of creativity and collaboration, individual autonomy and decentralized decison-making, which are all the characteristics of empowerment, along with a strong commitment to in-service training for all those involved. In this study we see the rejection of the power-coercive and rational–empirical approaches in favour of the bottom-up and empowering normative–re-educative approach to change.

In writing about how individuals are affected by the change process, Davis concludes that this must involve recognition by management of the individual's need to be self-empowering, while individuals must recognize the need to be resilient and reflective in their practice, seeing change as a learning experience.

Another educationalist who has investigated the effects of the Project 2000 changes is Jill Robinson (1991) and she too has gone to the work of Marris as a key source, citing his view that there is a characteristic resistance and ambivalence to change which is necessary as part of the adaptation process needed for survival (Marris, 1984). This view sees humans as needing a frame of reference, built up over the years from our own experiences, against which new stimuli can be compared and hence made sense of. This is similar to how social psychologists see the development of attitudes and helps explain our natural resistance to change. The experiences of Hunt (1987) in trying to introduce change but failing because staff felt anxious and uncertain about the changes in practice involved immediately spring to mind (p. 74).

Robinson argues therefore that resistance to change is not automatically all bad; rather it is a means of coping with change and finding meaning within the new situation. Ambivalence should therefore be recognized for what it is, a coping mechanism, and consequently tolerated and worked through progressively. Dissonance theory predicts a gradual shift in attitude with time which will steadily encompass the changed world in a more positive way. This approach is also consistent with the views of Marris as it permits individuals slowly to make sense of their new environment and get their bearings, in the process feeling more secure and less anxious. Most nurses can remember their first day on a new ward and the fears and anxieties that generated, yet after 2 months, when they felt they knew their way around, going on duty provoked nothing like the same fear and anxiety. We would do well to reflect upon and learn from our own experiences!

An example of an action-research approach to change in the field of mental health is provided by the work of Armitage *et al.* (1991). These workers studied two continuing care wards where the approaches to care were described as outmoded, custodial and with little or no attempt at rehabilitation. The aim was to implement primary nursing as a means of improving the quality of care given.

The researchers realized very early on that staff displayed signs reminiscent of Seligman's famous work on learned helplessness (1975). As a result of experience they had become used to being undervalued, passive and with little control over what went on around them. They had learned to be helpless. Efforts were made therefore to engage the staff in small-scale changes just to show change was possible and that their views mattered. This involved the staff in the research and began a process of empowerment. Conscious efforts were made to raise the profile of the wards within the hospital pecking order from their previous 'back ward' status in order to improve staff morale further and it was possible to carry out some building and decorating works to improve the general ward environment.

The study achieved a modest degree of success in that primary nursing was successfully implemented and key indicators showed significant improvements in care. The outcomes will be reviewed later in Chapter 7; what matters for now is rather the approaches that were used to implement change. The use of action research coupled with a participative style is important. The author's discussion of staff who had learned to be helpless is striking and their work in empowering the staff seems to have been a key ingredient in achieving the modest success they did. Work done on improving the physical environment was considered important also. The authors point out that, although the change achieved was modest, it was made with the regular ward staff, which suggests that the changes that have occurred have a better chance of remaining in place, rather than being carried out by staff specially brought in for the project who then leave.

This study shows obstacles to change being removed (improving the environment, getting rid of low morale, removing the ward's low status) whilst positive forces driving change forwards were introduced, such as empowering the staff and the presence of the action-research workers. This study therefore fits the Lewin force field theory of change and shows considerable evidence of a bottom-up approach and staff empowerment. It is suggested therefore that this example shows that change for the better is possible in even the most unpromising circumstances, providing certain key principles are adhered to.

Another interesting view of mental health nursing and change comes from the work of Massey (1991) who hypothesized that nurses working in large mental hospitals facing closure might experience an anticipatory grief reaction which he termed institutional loss. This is consistent with the views of Kotter and Schlesinger (1986) who suggest that staff involved in change may experience a sense of loss. Massey investigated a small sample of 22 nurses, 13 of whom were still working in what had been a large institution (the Mendip Hospital near Wells in Somerset) and 9 of whom had moved out from the Mendip into community settings. He was looking for evidence of mourning and anticipatory grief which he claimed to find in the data. It has to be said, however, that the samples were very small and not subject therefore to statistical analysis, while the work can be criticized from the point of view that the researcher set out looking for something and found it – this raises the question of unintentional bias.

This study is of importance for several reasons despite these methodological difficulties. It points to an area which will affect many nurses (and clients) in the rest of this decade with the move to community care, and not just in the field of mental health and learning disability as large general hospitals are also facing closure as a result of population shifts and the switch to a market-driven NHS. This study merits replication with a larger sample which will permit statistical testing of the significance of the findings.

If community care is to be successful, nursing staff must enter the field with a positive attitude and a willingness to work in the new system. Should nursing enter this arena with a negative attitude and fail to make the case for nursing care in the community, then nursing will be doing itself and the clients a grave disservice. There is a real risk that much nursing care will be taken over by social services, resulting in a situation whereby social workers and health-care assistants assume the roles more correctly taken by professional nurses. It is therefore essential that this change is handled constructively and that nursing shows what excellent results it can really achieve in the community rather than resisting change.

If institutional loss is a valid concept, this will be a handicap to nursing, hence the importance of further research into the area and an approach to change that is sensitive to the issues that have been outlined in this chapter. Nurses facing the closure of their hospital have little choice in their future nursing role. Dissonance theory suggests therefore that movement to the community must be accompanied by the perception of substantial reward in the new forms of working if the nurse is to adopt a more positive attitude to community care. Those responsible for such areas of nursing might reflect upon the way community care is presented to staff therefore as emphasis upon improvements and the positive rewards associated with such moves might facilitate a more positive staff attitude. A participative, bottom-up approach will also have much to commend it if the goal of management is a strong community nursing service. But is it? There is a strong antinursing, antiprofessionalism streak amongst some NHS managers introduced into the market-driven NHS of the 1990s.

The value of involving staff in the change process and thereby empowering them is shown by an investigation into that most thorny of issues, ward atmosphere. This study was carried out by James *et al.* (1990) in a unit within a large learning disability hospital. The researchers used the ward atmosphere scale (WAS) developed by Moos (1974) which measures staff views about the ideal and actual state of interpersonal relationships, treatment programmes and system maintenance within any therapeutic environment.

A total of 26 staff were involved (12 of whom were nursing auxiliaries) and this group was divided into two groups. All staff completed the questionnaire twice to provide a stable baseline measure of how they perceived the atmosphere on the ward and against which to measure subsequent change. Staff completed the questionnaire a total of five times during the research period, the key difference being that one group was merely given individual written feedback on score progress while the other group met for group discussions concerning the ward and the scores on the questionnaires. Members of this latter group were therefore involved participants who felt they had a say in how the ward was running.

The results showed that, although there were no significant differences between the groups at the start, by the end of the study, those involved in active feedback and discussion concerning the ward atmosphere were rating the social environment significantly more favourably than those who were not and who only received individual written feedback. The researchers conclude that the WAS is a useful tool for assessing ward atmosphere and also for providing staff with the sort of structured information that can help change it, providing the staff are all actively involved in such discussions.

This study again demonstrates the value of empowering staff by participation within group settings and moving away from hierarchical models. The authors note cautiously, however, that they cannot guarantee that the positive changes generated by this intervention will persist as their study only covered a 6-month period. They underline the importance of freezing the change by ensuring that the factors which brought it about are incorporated within the new system.

Conclusion

The examples referred to above demonstrate that the key ingredients for change outlined in this chapter are found to be present when successful change occurs. They may be summarized as:

- A bottom-up approach, maximizing staff participation.
- Sensitivity to staff anxieties and fears.
- Avoiding top-down direction and coercion.
- Not relying solely on rational logic.
- Attitude change.
- Loose structures, a bias for action, avoiding bureaucracy.
- Empowerment.
- Critical reflection on practice.
- Education as a means of liberation.
- Leadership which, amongst other qualities, is sensitive to and acknowledges the importance of the above factors.

This is by no means an exhaustive list but should be considered as some of the key items whose presence will facilitate change.

It is important to look at change from the individual's point of view at all times and to see initial resistance as a normal part of the way we adapt to change. It is worth therefore considering an important observation made by Fitzgerald (1991) who cautions nurses against paying too much attention to the strategy of change at the expense of the content of change, i.e. nursing itself. Theory can only underpin practice as long as it is relevant to practice. This is a key observation in considering strategies for changing nursing: how relevant are such strategies to nursing? Just because some high-powered executive from the world of commerce feels he knows the secret of change, we should not accept these views without asking how relevant such theories are to nursing.

Finally, it should now be possible to address the paradox of nursing and change. The reason nursing appears to resist change most of the time and yet be subject to sudden overnight changes is that they are usually imposed using the power-coercion top-down model. This gives the appearance of change taking place quickly, but in reality little has changed as people generally resent such approaches to change and largely carry on as before. The gulf that exists between NHS management and clinical nurses is such that management probably do not even realize that little change has occurred in practice. The only change they understand is names on pieces of paper and sums on the ledger pages (or computer printouts, to be more up to date); consequently, all change effort is directed towards these areas at the expense of something that management do not understand – nursing and patient care.

The lack of real change in nursing therefore can be seen as stemming from a failure to approach change from the perspectives outlined above. Instead we are locked into our hierarchical culture which is about power, status and coercion. Cultures are very difficult to change, as we have seen, and the present culture of the NHS and nursing blocks nurse-led changes in patient care while rushing ahead with grand organizational changes which are ideologically and financially driven. Education is the key to undermining this cultural straitjacket, along with the recognition by nurses that they actually are an oppressed group and do not have to be so. Critical social theory suggests that nurses can change the system and reclaim nursing for nurses.

References

Armitage P, Champney-Smith J, Andrews K (1991) Primary nursing and the role of the preceptor in changing long term mental health care: an evaluation. *Journal of Advanced Nursing* **16**: 413–422.

Benner P (1984) *From Novice to Expert*. New York, Addison Wesley.

Davis P (1991) The meaning of change to individuals within a college of nurse education. *Journal of Advanced Nursing* **16**: 108–115.

Driscoll S (1982) Nurses and the change process. *New Zealand Nursing Journal* **75**: 3–4.

FitzGerald M (1991) Making things happen. *Nursing Times* **87**: 30, 25–27.

Franklin B (1758) *Poor Richard's Almanac*.

Freire P (1985) *The Politics of Education; Culture, Power and Liberation*. New York, Macmillan.

Gleick J (1987) *Chaos*. New York, Cardinal.

Griffiths R (1985) *Inquiry into NHS Management*. London, Department of Health.
Hunt M (1987) The process of translating research findings into nursing practice. *Journal of Advanced Nursing* **12**: 101–110.
James, I, Milne D, Firth H (1990) A systematic comparison of feedback and staff discussion in changing the ward atmosphere. *Journal of Advanced Nursing* **15**: 329–336.
Kotter J, Schlesinger L (1986) Choosing strategies for change. In: Maynon-White W (ed) *Planning and Managing Change*. London, Harper & Row.
Lewin K (1951) *Field Theory in the Social Sciences*. New York, Harper.
Lupton T (1986) Organisational change; top down or bottom up management. In: Maynon-White W (ed) *Planning and Managing Change*. London, Harper & Row.
Marris P (1975) *Loss and Change*. London, Routledge & Kegan Paul.
Massey P (1991) Institutional loss: an examination of a bereavement reaction in 22 mental nurses losing their institution and moving into the community. *Journal of Advanced Nursing* **16**: 573–583.
Moos RH (1974) *Evaluating Treatment Environments*. New York, Wiley.
Peters T, Waterman R (1986) A bias for action. In: Maynon-Whyte W (ed) *Planning and Managing Change*. London, Harper & Row.
Robinson J (1991) Project 2000: the role of resistance in the process of professional growth. *Journal of Advanced Nursing* **16**: 820–824.
Rogers E, Shoemaker F (1971) *Communication of Innovations: A Cross Cultural Report*, 2nd edn. New York, Free Press.
Seligman M (1975) *Helplessness. On Development, Depression and Death*. San Francisco, Freeman.
Sheehan J (1990) Investigating change in a nursing context. *Journal of Advanced Nursing* **15**: 819–824.
Stroebe W, Jonas K (1988) Strategies and attitude change. In: Hewstone M (ed) *Introduction to Social Psychology*. Oxford, Blackwell.
Towell D, Harries C (1979) *Innovation in Patient Care: An Action Research Study of Change in a Psychiatric Hospital*. London, Croom Helm.
Walsh M, Ford P (1989) *Nursing Rituals: Research and Rational Action*. Butterworth-Heinemann, Oxford
Webb C (1989) Action research: philosophy, methods and personal experiences. *Journal of Advanced Nursing* **14**: 403–410.
Williams A, Dobson P, Walters M (1989) *Changing Culture*. London, Institute of Personnel Managers.

5 *Liberation nursing*

Stone walls do not a prison make
  Nor iron bars a cage;
Minds innocent and quiet take
  That for an hermitage;
If I have freedom in my love,
  And in my soul am free;
Angels alone, that soar above,
  Enjoy such liberty.
                    Richard Lovelace (1618–1658) *To Althea, from Prison*

The need for liberation implies imprisonment and loss of freedom. Nursing today faces precisely this problem but, as Richard Lovelace's words suggest, freedom and liberty may be achieved even within the constraining environment of the market-driven NHS, if within nursing itself we are free.

Nursing is held in thrall by a range of internal and external forces. Powerful external forces involving the balance of power have maintained nursing in a subordinate role to the medical profession and, increasingly within the last few years, to the general management élite and their political masters. The absence of a home-grown nursing knowledge base (until recently), due to its externally controlled dependence upon medicine and other disciplines, has prevented professional autonomy from developing. The emphasis placed on positivist scientific knowledge has devalued attempts to build a nursing knowledge base and exacerbated this problem. To be free requires independence of thought and knowledge.

The de-skilling, antiprofessional agenda being followed by senior management since the removal of nurse managerial autonomy in the aftermath of the Griffiths Report is a prime example of the way nursing is having its freedom eroded. This is underscored by the use of contractual gagging clauses which remove the basic human right of freedom of speech from nurses and other staff. A more subtle restriction has been the media portrayal of nurses as obedient handmaidens, mindless bimbos and sex objects, none of which are conducive to a role involving autonomy and freedom and all of which have contributed to the subordination of nursing by dominant groups such as managers and the medical profession.

Such portrayals are as much a ball and chain around nursing's ankle as any dinosaur the medical profession may produce.

Internal forces stem from history and the culture of hierarchy and obedience; this latter point is exacerbated by gender stereotyping. Such a culture is difficult to alter and will itself serve to impede change which moves in the direction of empowerment. Traditional nurse training and a careful selection policy of recruits who will not rock the boat, rather than a truly challenging and stimulating education, have also contributed to the propagation of the status quo. The absence of nursing research until recently is another factor that has limited nursing's freedom to develop. When practice becomes a prisoner of dogma rather than based upon factual knowledge, we are indeed reminded that stone walls do not a prison make.

Nursing has much to do within its own boundaries, in addition to facing the challenges from external oppressors. The freedom to nurse is being removed from nurses by NHS management who wish to replace it with their own élitist, managerial culture. Understanding little if anything of care, they seek instead to turn carers into managers of care, devaluing the nature of care in the process to the level of something that a person with a basic schooling and some on-the-job, task-based, National Vocational Qualification (NVQ) training can accomplish. This devaluation of caring comes in the wake of the New Right critique of what is dubbed the 'dependency culture' of the 1970s and the individualistic, selfish decade of the 1980s which resulted from the ascendancy of the New Right in politics. Caring has been one of the main casualties of the 1980s.

There are many within the management élite who argue that this is just traditional trade union protectionism, nurses defending the jobs of nurses. That in itself is no sin, although a more robust response might be that it is nurses defending the rights of the general public to have access to skilled professional care, providing of course that such care is indeed skilled and professional rather than traditional procedure-manual dogma. It is relevant to ask whether managers who level such charges of protectionism against nurses apply the same standards to themselves. Might there not be occasions when some managers are guilty of empire-building themselves? If there was a consensus view that the care offered by the NHS had increased proportionally with the increase in management staff, and there was a direct link between the two, then that increase might be justifiable. Outside of government and

NHS management circles there is little agreement with any such proposition, so how can managers as a class justify their high salaries and growth in numbers at the expense of 'hands-on' NHS workers? The charge of protectionism might better be levelled at managers in this case. It is sad that managerial empires are being built at the expense of patient care and nursing freedom.

It is time for nurses to reclaim nursing as an act of caring and in the process break free from the imprisoning walls of management diktat while we still have the power to do so. There are large-scale political battles to fight with government over the future of the NHS and nursing's place within it. The nurse may be forgiven for considering such targets as Secretaries of State and Department of Health Committees as remote and inaccessible, which of course is no coincidence. However, professional bodies and unions such as the Royal College of Nursing (RCN) and the United Kingdom Central Council for Nursing, Midwifery and Health Visiting (UKCC) do have the resources to make their voices heard in such quarters, and with the active support of more nurses could make their voices even louder. The RCN in particular has been vigorously defending nursing's position while the Royal College of Midwives has been advancing the cause of midwifery. Would that more nurses and midwives joined the still small band of activists within such organizations! Nurses should also remember that government ministers do have to go cap in hand to the country every 4 or 5 years for re-election and nurses collectively have a large number of votes to use. Political action can be both direct as well as indirect.

However, there are more accessible targets which are amenable to change every day of the week and this is what the rest of this chapter is about. Nurses do not need to wait for a general election or a major national campaign by the RCN to attack the internal forces which constrain and subordinate nursing. We have it within our power to move away from hierarchical nursing structures and open up ward and community teams to a more equal, empowering style of working. First must come the recognition that the traditional view of power is only one view, a peculiarly male view; there are others, as we have seen already, which rely on sharing and consensus to empower all members of the nursing team and in the process liberate them from authoritarian control.

Critical social theory encourages nurses to recognize their suppression and consequently to act themselves to assert control over their own lives and professional practice. Nurses should not wait for heroes and liberators; messiahs have a habit of often turning out to be false; rather it is about nurses empowering each other collectively to liberate nursing. Empowerment however is a concept that is equally valid for patients. Nurses must extend and develop the work that is going on in empowering patients, as in this way they empower themselves.

Managers may try and gag nurses from talking about what they do, but NHS trusts have not yet introduced Orwellian thought police to stop nurses thinking about their practice. This leaves open the opportunity for nurses to develop into reflective practitioners and in the process, value more truly the work they do. Not only will thinking about what we do and why we do it lead to improved ways of working, but collection of such knowledge will help make visible much of the currently invisible quality work that nurses carry out and develop a knowledge base for caring independent of the biomedical model. A nursing grown from its roots in everyday practice is unlikely to be led up blind alleys by charismatic individuals or high-powered promotional companies with glossy leaflets. Reflection upon and during practice will instead liberate the nurse from the ritualistic dogma of the procedure manual.

Nurse educationalists have it within their power to educate nurses for freedom. The introduction of the Project 2000 reforms and the steady growth of pre-registration undergraduate nursing courses, coupled with exciting post-registration opportunities such as the English Nursing Board Higher Award and a range of part-time nursing diploma and degree courses, can all act as a powerful engine which will drive nursing towards liberation from the outmoded training-based past we have inherited. Education must equip nurses with the critical faculties to discern between good new ideas and new ideas that only sound good but will turn into tomorrow's dogma and ritual.

Education can lead to nothing short of revolution, but it can also be used to preserve the status quo as critical social theorists have eloquently argued. Educators can give nurses the tools to break free from the chains of ritual and tradition and also to defend nursing against those managers who would replace nursing education with a task-based, NVQ training philosophy.

One key area that educationalists can drive forwards is that of developing a research base for nursing knowledge as the ability to carry out research has to be learnt like anything else. Nursing should, however, beware the trap of following the path of one of the dominant groups, medicine, and seeing research as only a positivist, empirical, number-crunching activity. That will imprison nursing in the same way that looking at the world through half-closed eyes will, as there is much more to see and discover beyond the discipline of hypothesis and statistical significance. Standing on top of Blencathra in Cumbria looking south gives the impression the Lake District is about wide open green valleys, a small town (Keswick) and a busy trunk road (A66). Turn and face the other way and the wilderness of Carrock Fell stretches away for miles – a totally different impression. So it is with research, for if nurses employ more qualitative and action-research-based methods they will uncover areas of knowledge hitherto inaccessible. Just as a true picture of any landscape will only be seen by looking in all directions, so it is with nursing: all the different research traditions should be employed, not just one.

Change is a key component of liberation and there is much that can be changed within nursing regardless of management; this is part of the process of reclaiming nursing for nurses. The preceding chapter showed, though, that there are many pitfalls in the way of change and argued for change to be carried out in a participative, bottom-up style that paid particular attention to individuals' attitudes, beliefs and anxieties. Some essential characteristics of liberating change are given on p. 81. Relating the last point to this one, it is essential to show that change, once implemented, actually makes a difference; this underlines the importance of research, particularly action research. The argument for nursing praxis, the changing of nursing through practice, can only be won if nurses can demonstrate that innovation makes a positive difference to outcome.

A rider must be added to this statement, however – for in considering outcomes we must ask: 'Whose outcomes?'. Various groups of people will be affected by outcomes in different ways and thus perceive outcomes differently. Outcomes can be measured in terms of the patient, the nurse or the system. A change may be shown as making the patient happier, but if other parts of the system are unhappy with that change, for example, one group of staff within the system feel it infringes their prerogative or another group feel it costs too much, then however beneficial the change might be to the patient, there are powerful others who will block it. Nurses must not be naïve and assume that because they can demonstrate a positive patient outcome, this will guarantee successful nurse-led change. Unfortunately, this is not enough. The nurse has to be politically astute enough to see who else is involved and in researching the case for change take these other factors into account.

A final characteristic of liberation nursing is perhaps stating the obvious but is none the less important for that – it must provide choice for both patient and nurse. If the nurse or patient has no choice in what is happening, no influence over decisions, then they cannot be said to be free. The 1992 UKCC document *Scope of Professional Practice* is a welcome example of choice for this did away with the restrictive constraints of the 'extended role of the nurse' policy. Nurses may now choose, in the light of their own expertise, how to develop their practice without internal nursing-imposed limitations. In making this change the UKCC have shown that nursing can make changes which do liberate nursing. It is to be hoped that they will not stop here, however, and go on to develop a more robust profile in the future to defend nursing freedom.

The concept of extending choice means there must also be a fundamental rethink about nurse–patient relationships, for example, as the traditional doctor/nurse-knows-best approach is no longer acceptable. If nurses wish to be empowered and free themselves in their practice, so too must patients be free to choose when it comes to treatment and care delivery.

The view of liberation nursing expressed here is of something that questions and challenges authoritarian power structures, preferring instead to empower nurses by consensus and collaboration. This process must be extended to patients. Reflection upon practice is seen as a crucial element in developing nursing knowledge and expertise while education is advocated as a means of freeing nursing from the traditions, rituals and constraints of both the past and present. The discovery of fresh knowledge through a range of research approaches which should be close to the patient/nurse caring relationship can only give nursing more ammunition in its struggle for professional freedom. Change within nursing is possible providing key guidelines are followed that avoid the traps associated with the authoritarian models of power that nursing should now reject.

Nursing still has the authority to free itself from the past and to build a professional body of expertise that will ensure its survival and growth as a strong, independent profession. This dynamic approach requires major changes in how nursing is carried out if the struggle to liberate nursing from its hierarchical and ritualistic past, let alone the controls and shackles of the present, is to succeed. The phrase *liberation nursing* is suggested as a means of expressing this approach to care and some key components are summarized below. Liberation nursing should:

- Value individual patients/nurses and their freedom of choice and speech.
- Encourage maximum participation by all who have something to contribute whilst removing hierarchies from the care system.
- Value and develop reflective practice.
- Be based upon a range of research strategies.
- Give the nurse the confidence to work towards equal partner ship with the patient (patient empowerment).
- Utilize education as a means of liberating practice.
- Show a bias towards flexibility and change whilst recognizing the meaning of change to the individual.
- Value the expertise of the clinical nurse.
- Strive to achieve praxis, i.e. change practice by the process of doing.

There are those who would imprison nursing for the sake of adding to their own power or pursuing a political ideology. The evocative words of Richard Lovelace that opened this chapter should remind nurses that collectively and individually we have freedom in our love of nursing. Nursing has a 'soul': it is that set of humanitarian, caring values that is characteristic of nursing, and within that 'soul' we are free. The unconscious irony of the use of the word 'angels' in Lovelace's work will not be lost on the reader, but nursing can emulate the last two lines of his poem by developing an empowering, liberating strategy for action which in the future will allow nursing to soar above the entrenched attitudes and political dogma. Is the opposition nursing faces today any greater than that facing Miss Nightingale in the previous century?

This liberating approach to nursing has little truck with élitism, power structures, hierarchies, gagging clauses that prohibit freedom of speech and the reductionism that breaks care down into a series of unrelated, conveyor-belt tasks. In the next section a range of recent nursing initiatives will be examined to see how effectively they may liberate nursing. The ideas discussed in this first section of the book and summarized above will be used as litmus paper to test their liberating potential. However, where there is a danger of intro-ducing new rituals for old, nursing must recognize that danger if it is to avoid imprisoning itself within a professional straitjacket whilst simultaneously succumbing to the increasing domination of non-nursing groups who are pursuing their own agendas of power.

Reference

UKCC (1992) *Scope of Professional Practice*. London, UKCC.

PART TWO

The Delivery
of Care

In this section we will examine some of the key concepts which have appeared in nursing in the last decade or so which impact upon the delivery of nursing care. Our purpose is not to show that research supports this idea or rejects that idea. Nursing is too complex for such straightforward answers. Rather, we are using the ideas and theories explored in Part One to test the strengths and weaknesses of these new nursing concepts. Research findings are important, but so too is probing with questions and the examination of the implications of some of the big new ideas. Only by asking awkward questions and working through the consequences of new concepts can we avoid sheepishly following the false messiahs and work towards the liberation of nursing.

6 *Questions of quality*

Introduction

Is quality assurance work a crucial aspect of care that offers nurses a great opportunity to promote and liberate our profession or is it, as Allen (1991) suggested, becoming merely a cliché? Similar doubts led Shelley (1992) to wonder if the topic had become just another trendy bandwagon that everybody was jumping on. Change in nursing must be for the better, which implies that those advocating new approaches to care such as primary nursing need to demonstrate that such initiatives improve the quality of nursing care delivered. There are therefore some crucial questions to be asked about quality.

Can quality assurance empower staff and patients or is it another management task, imposed from on high, carried out half-heartedly, which will degenerate into just another ritual? Do the various quality assurance methods measure what they say they measure and are they reliable? For all the assurances of the experts, do they actually measure the right things for, as Jane Austen wrote in *Sense and Sensibility*, 'Where so many hours have been spent in convincing myself that I am right, is there not some reason to fear that I may be wrong?' Is it even possible to 'assure' quality and what is quality anyway? Questions of quality such as these need to be explored before nurses become too embroiled in the plethora of quality assurance work that abounds today.

What is quality?

There are many answers to this fundamental question which must be addressed before discussion can proceed any further. Barnett (1992) approached this issue from a philosophical viewpoint. He suggests the word 'quality' is so subjective that it conveys little more than an inner positive feeling towards whatever entity is being discussed. It may therefore be given many meanings so that it tells us much more about the person using it than the element in question. Nurses should therefore beware simplistic definitions, for there is no objective, unique definition of quality; it means different things to different people.

The nursing profession, for example, has become obsessed with setting standards, yet this exercise appears at times to be little more than a modern version of demanding all the bed wheels be straight and all the pillow case openings face the same way (away from the door!). Unthinking regimentation is but a short step away from setting standards.

The subjective nature of quality is developed by Barnett in considering the three principal approaches to defining quality that may be found in the literature. He argues that any public service is subject to three sets of influences which stem from the practitioners in the field, government and the consumers (market forces). Practitioners tend to favour peer-review methods of ensuring quality (quality circles, the Royal College of Nursing Dynamic Standard Setting System (DySSSy) method), government agencies look to performance indicators and outcome measures, whilst market-led influences will generate consumer-led approaches such as client satisfaction ratings. These three approaches pull against each other and lead to rival definitions of quality.

The situation might be simplified by suggesting that there are two basic approaches discernible within this model. First, there is an internal approach where practitioners define quality according to their own values, which assumes of course that the practitioners know best. Alternatively there is an outside, instrumental approach where consumers and government agencies define quality. Their points of departure are values which may well differ from the professional values of practitioners; their route of travel involves inputs and outputs, costs and benefits; their right to pronounce on the issue derives from being consumers or paymasters.

Nurses are increasingly finding themselves caught between these differing approaches as they may want to develop a home-grown, bottom-up approach to quality but NHS trust boards are responding to contract specifications that reflect the government's priorities, such as the Patient's Charter and the targets set out in the *Health of the Nation*.

Wherever the statements of quality come from, they are usually expressed in terms of standards or levels of performance which should be achieved. Measurements are then carried out to see how successful staff are in achieving these standards. The focus is therefore upon a quantitative approach. This has two serious implications which have been identified by Koch (1992). First, if nurses do not have the skills to carry out what is effectively sophisticated research, particularly with regard to concepts of measurement, the result will be poor-quality data which will fail to influence nursing care for the better. Her second point is that all this work is ignoring what the patient understands and experiences as nursing care. Meaningful information about the patient's subjective perceptions is left out of the quality equation. Perhaps we could paraphrase that well-known nursing phrase and ponder upon the assertion that the quality of care is what the patient says it is.

Should professional nurses alone set standards? They would be accused of being paternalistic if they claimed that quality should be left to them alone to determine without outside interference. Yorke (1992) has on the other hand argued that too heavy an external evaluation of quality by senior management and government agencies runs the risk of a compliance culture wherein practitioners are so busy demonstrating that they can meet externally set targets that key areas of a team's philosophy may be subverted and lost. Patient throughput goals may be achieved but the philosophy of individualized holistic care may have gone out of the window in the process, while nobody thinks to check the readmission rates, which might be associated with impressive throughput statistics.

Of course, it is not as simple as this in the real world as there are many areas of overlap where different groups ask similar questions, but Barnett's central argument remains valid for all that – quality holds different meanings and is therefore to be measured in different ways, depending upon who is asking the questions. It is a very complex phenomenon, an amalgam of concepts and a coupling of philosophical and sociological perspectives which Barnett has described as more a babel of voices than a debate. Simple it is not.

Quality, validity and reliability

If nurses are to seek to measure the quality of care by any of the three broad approaches introduced above, two crucial aspects of the exercise are the validity and reliability of the methods used. Discussion of these concepts stems usually from texts on research methodology and, as we have argued elsewhere in this book, a lack of understanding about research has been a major handicap for nursing in the past. Reliability and validity are not abstract concepts best left to the academics; they are too important for that. Any nurse thinking about quality, or reading about or embarking upon research, must have a working knowledge of these concepts. A moment's reflection should show that any quality work is research in itself, as it involves the discovery of knowledge. Quality assurance that ignores reliability and validity issues is meaningless.

Reliability refers to consistency and accuracy whilst validity means the extent to which something measures what it says it is measuring. Something can therefore be reliable, but not valid. A tape measure can reliably measure your inside-leg measurement, i.e. consistently get the same answer when measurements are repeated several times by different people, an answer which we can be confident is correct by checking with several other tape measures. However, this is not a valid measurement of your ability to pass exams and successfully complete academic courses! The tape measure is a reliable measure of your inside leg but not a valid measure of your academic ability.

Reliability is probably the easier of these two concepts to check and understand. For example, if quality is being measured by observation, it is essential to have two independent observers separately recording what they see. Their scores can then be compared after the observation period and correlated. A high degree of correlation promotes confidence that they are both correct; however, it also means they could be equally wrong – an important possibility that is often overlooked. A low correlation between scores indicates serious observational error by at least one person and, as it is not usually possible to tell which, the information from both observers is therefore deemed unreliable.

Correlations can only work if there is a sense of order or degree in what is being observed, such as, for example, scores on the Waterlow pressure sore risk scale. If instead the observer is counting the frequency with which things are done, i.e. categories of behaviour such as talking to patients, this is known as categorical data and cannot be correlated in the usual way. The two observers count the frequencies of the observed behaviour or completed documentation, for example, and express their scores as a ratio. The closer it is to 1, the better the agreement and the more reliable the observation is said to be. However there is a problem here also; a certain number of agreements would occur by chance alone;

therefore the ratio derived is falsely optimistic. Correction for chance agreement is needed and Everitt and Hay (1992) demonstrate how this may be done by use of the kappa statistic.

Validity is not so amenable to checking. The sort of question that should be asked is to what extent is a box ticked on a questionnaire which asks the patient to rate satisfaction with care actually measuring how satisfied the patient really is with care? Do the scores derived from objective measures such as Qualpacs or Monitor really represent the quality of care given, or do they represent something else? Koch (1992) argues very strongly, for example, that the complexity of care is such that it cannot be captured by numbers alone, while Balogh (1992) argues that not one of the various quality-measuring tools has had its validity demonstrated in the UK.

How then is validity demonstrated? One common way is to show that a tool is based upon another well-used tool. This is fraught with dangers because who is to say that the original tool is valid? The Rush Medicus Instrument from which Monitor was developed is based upon the nursing process and derives validity from this source, but where is the evidence that the nursing process is a valid method of delivering high-quality nursing care? Chapter 9 explores this issue further.

The adaptation process may itself threaten and undermine validity. Moving an instrument to another culture or country may destroy its validity. By analogy, a person may hold a valid gun licence in the USA but may not carry a weapon in the UK with the same licence, just as a car which is judged fit for the road in Manchester, Massachusetts may not be judged fit by the Greater Manchester constabulary, UK. Validity does not automatically cross the Atlantic; it has to be demonstrated afresh.

An alternative approach is referred to as criterion validity. Polit and Hungler (1987) define this concept in terms of the strength of the relationship in scores between a new measure and an existing, already validated measure. The old measure is therefore used as a yardstick or criterion to test the new. If there is a good correlation between scores, criterion validity is said to be demonstrated.

To demonstrate the criterion validity of any of the methods used to measure quality in the UK, it would be necessary to show that their scores correlate with another measure, or criterion which measures quality. As Balogh (1992) has shown, attempts at correlating scores using various combinations of quality-measuring tools have all failed. Evidence for the criterion validity of quality-measuring instruments is lacking. Balogh concludes from this that quality is multidimensional; it cannot be measured with only one scale. Such a one-track approach lacks validity.

Consider being given a bucket of paint and the task of describing and measuring it. A tape measure would allow description of its size and dimensions, a weighing scale its weight, a measuring jug its volume, and a colour chart its precise colour. Already we need four different measurement scales and we have not begun to measure its viscosity or find out whether it is suitable for indoor or outdoor use. If at least six different measures are needed to describe a bucket of paint, how many are needed to describe the quality of something so complex as nursing care?

This brief section has introduced the ideas of reliability and validity which are crucial to any meaningful understanding of quality measurement. These concepts will recur later in this chapter. The key point is that we should not accept the reliability or validity of any method that purports to measure quality of nursing care without insisting upon a demonstration of these characteristics.

The three principal approaches to quality which were introduced at the start of this chapter will now be critiqued, not only with issues of reliability and validity in mind, but also to ask whether they are empowering and liberating concepts.

Objective and generic measuring tools

Preformulated tools meant to assess care in general rather than any specific speciality are very attractive as somebody else has done all the hard work of setting the standards and designing the instrument. They also give scores which have the beguiling appearance of being easy to understand and are consequently every manager's dream. It is to these that we will turn our attention first.

Government and NHS management have a lengthy history of being interested in estimating the size of the nursing work-force required to deliver any given standard of care. Researchers have typically tried to divide patients up into various categories of dependence and look at the tasks that nurses perform to try and arrive at a match between the two. This approach has been much criticized as it paints a very narrow picture of nursing – the crucial psychosocial elements are omitted, for example.

This 'scientific' approach to investigating nursing work reached its peak in the view of Balogh (1992) with the Aberdeen formula for calculating staffing requirements which was based upon patient dependence categories and timings of nursing care carried out on a group of wards where nursing care was judged to reach acceptable standards. The criteria for 'acceptable standards' are very vague, which seriously weakens this work.

The Aberdeen formula was discredited by the work of Gault (1982), who re-examined the original data (gathered in 1969) and showed that it was statistically flawed. The conclusions reached by the original proponents of the model were untenable when the data on which they were based were subjected to rigorous statistical scrutiny. Analysis of the data showed that what nurses did with their time depended upon the amount of time they had available, rather than some artificially constructed model based upon patient dependence. Gault was critical of assumptions that had been made about causality in how nurses utilized their time and of the way the original study had ignored nurses' professional judgement of situations which influenced how they spent time. Time did not appear to correspond to any patient dependence classification, which suggests that the classifications lacked meaning and validity or that the pursuit of ward routine was at the expense of highly dependent patients. The date of this study has to be remembered – 1969, when it may be assumed that the wards in question were largely run on traditional, task-oriented lines.

Various attempts have followed the Aberdeen formula right up to the present day in trying to calculate staffing levels that will deliver an 'acceptable standard of care'. According to Balogh (1992), they all suffer from problems, the most obvious of which is that results from one location do not translate automatically into another care setting. This non-transference leads to a great deal of work as non-nurse managers who will not trust nursing judgement require repeated measurements or staff find themselves with inappropriate measures foisted upon them. We have already mentioned that these measures are usually insensitive to the psychosocial dimensions of care and there is also frequently confusion over the purpose of the exercise: establishment-setting and staff allocation are two different things. Perhaps the biggest problem of all is inability to build quality into the equation and decide just what is an acceptable standard of care and how that may be measured and monitored. What is acceptable to management may not be acceptable to nursing staff.

It is this management-led need for quantifiable data that has led to the growth of a range of audit tools and scoring systems which seek to express quality in terms of numbers. We would argue that nursing care is too complex for such an approach. Although there are advantages in producing objective measures of quality, it is only one dimension of care; the quality of nursing care cannot be reduced simply to numbers. As Koch (1992) has pointed out, nursing is complex, intimately linked to the changing context within which it occurs and reacts, and ultimately is beyond measurement. The interaction of the environment with the characteristics of the individual patient and nurse produces an infinite range of possibilities which are simply too complex to be captured in a simplistic checklist approach.

One of the earliest attempts at quantifying quality was the Phaneuf Nursing Audit, developed in the early 1960s in the USA. This system involves checking the documentation of a sample of patients, after discharge, at regular intervals using a 50-item checklist. There is an immediate validity problem with this approach: is checking documents actually checking quality of care? There would seem to be many situations in which the two could bear little relationship to each other. The scale is therefore not measuring what it says it is measuring, and so lacks validity.

Much better known in the UK is the Monitor system and its derivative, Senior Monitor, which is intended for use in elderly care settings. Monitor is a UK adaptation of the Rush Medicus quality monitoring methodology for nursing care. Kemp and Richardson (1990) summarize the instrument as following the nursing process methodology – a possible problem that has already been noted. It consists of six main objective areas, 32 subobjectives and a master (*sic*) criteria list of 357 items. From this massive bank of items, observer worksheets are generated which require some 30–50 items to be completed by interview and observation and then scored. A wide range of information sources involving patients, nurses and documentation is required.

Tomalin *et al.* (1992) have provided a clear account of the use of the Monitor system and have outlined a series of practical difficulties in its use. The layout of the booklet makes it difficult to have a realistic conversation with patients, for example, as the observer is continually moving from page to page to fill in relevant points. They could be far better grouped in a coherent fashion. There are difficulties in accessing data sources; nurses may be writing in the care plans so they are not available for scrutiny; the nurse required for interview may be busy, while the patient who should be interviewed may be off the ward or too ill to interview. Observation of care may require the assessor to intrude on intimate procedures, to the patient's embarrassment and therefore, ironically, may adversely affect the quality of care.

More serious than these practical difficulties are issues of reliability and validity. Some questions are ambiguous and many answers will be even more so, leading to difficulty with coding. This introduces problems of reliability because if the two observers have wide discrepancies in how they are coding answers to questions, the acid tests of consistency and accuracy will have been failed. Tomalin *et al.* stress the importance of observers spending time in advance of the exercise going through the questions and trying to agree how they will code certain answers, as well as again after the observation period, checking responses and trying to resolve differences of coding. The problem remains that this does not guarantee the accuracy of the exercise as both nurses could be equally wrong or if one nurse was a strong, dominant character, that individual's view may dominate consistently, introducing systematic bias. Substantial amounts of time should be allocated in order that the observation, coding and scoring work are optimally performed.

Even after adequate training, assessors may feel demoralized by the mechanistic nature of the work as it merely records the presence or absence of something and does not capture its essential quality. This raises the issue of validity again: is such an approach really measuring the quality of care? This point is underlined by Markham (1986) who reported that in using Monitor at the Royal Marsden, she was surprised to find that nursing staff only spend 6% of their time communicating with patients. The explanation given by Markham for this low figure is that time spent communicating with patients whilst performing other tasks, such as assisting with washing or dressing, was not recorded as communication. The tool therefore was not measuring what it said it was measuring and so its validity fails.

The issue raised by Koch (1992), that nursing is too complex to measure simply by numbers, returns again. The focus on measurement may override concerns about real care.

The construction of the instrument around the nursing process format means that any ward using patient-centred care is given a built-in advantage over more traditionally organized wards (Barnett and Wainwright, 1987). This should be borne in mind when Monitor or Senior Monitor is used as a research tool to investigate the effects of change from traditional nursing methods to new approaches such as primary nursing (see p. 148).

Despite this lengthy list of problems, Tomalin *et al.* feel it is possible to work around many of them with adequate experience, preparation and observer training. They also feel it is worth the effort, as Monitor does make staff question what they are doing and think about their care.

One further generic quality instrument of which many British nurses will have heard is the Qualpac system, which is based upon the Slater nursing performance rating scale. It is designed to be used by observing nursing in action over a list of 68 measures. Kemp and Richardson (1990) are critical of the ambiguity of some of the items and are very concerned at the amount of subjective judgement that is called for in making a quality assessment with Qualpacs. This clearly undermines the reliability of the tool. The validity of using the Qualpac system in the UK health-care setting is also questioned by these authors, although they acknowledge that, of the available scales, it is the one most concerned with how nurses react to patient needs. This strength has led Balogh (1992) to sound the cautionary note that, in a primary nursing ward, Qualpac puts each individual nurse's performance under the spotlight.

In addition to the type of quality tool, discussed above, which is concerned with nursing, nurses now have to live in the world of more general performance indicators, such as how many patients are treated per bed per year and at what cost? How valid a measure of quality are such indicators? As we shall see in Chapter 7, initiatives such as primary nursing mean that it will be possible for management to develop performance indicators for individual nurses. A primary nurse in the future may find the incidence of pressure sores or average length of stay in hospital of his/her patients being monitored and taken as an indication of performance, which of course could be linked to pay. The use of Qualpac, referred to above, makes this possible.

The new market orientation of the NHS is clearly driving much of this desire for numerical representations of quality, and with it constructing quality very differently from that which many nurses may wish. Evans and English (1992), for example, urge all managers and staff to understand quality in the same way and then go on to give a very autocratic managerial definition, 'conformance to

requirements', which begs the obvious question, whose requirements? This sounds very much like new 'NHS macho-manager
speak', especially when these writers go on to discuss quality as
being measured only in terms of money. To them quality is 'the cost
of doing things wrong.'

This approach totally ignores the consumer of health care – the
patient. The involvement of the patient and family in planning care
is a key dimension of quality. It is a very personal thing based upon
the individual's needs and desires. It certainly is not 'conformance
to requirements'.

Is it possible that these generic measurement tools will be of value
in the struggle to liberate nursing and empower patients? They offer
potential levers with which nursing may be able to prise more
resources from management but they also carry real dangers. The
language of these tools is the language that managers speak and, as
such, if nurses wish to engage in meaningful dialogue with the
power élite who dominate today's NHS, it is a language we have to
use. However, the validity of these generic tools is open to challenge
in the UK and urgent work needs to be done to establish that any
quality tool really is valid.

Norman *et al.* (1992) have reported on such an investigation
currently underway, in which they acknowledge that the claim of
objectivity is questionable and the reliability and validity shown
by these tools, when compared with each other in previous
studies, are low. These researchers are using the concept of
triangulation – measuring from different directions using different
methods to try and achieve convergence on the entity in question.
The goal is to try and confirm results by this approach and also to
ensure the completeness of what is under investigation – in this
case, the notion of quality and whether we really are fully
describing what is meant by this word. As these authors point out,
at present quality can mean almost anything, while high-quality
nursing care is a social construct which can be influenced by all
manner of things from ward to governmental level. There are
strong echoes of the philosophical introduction to this chapter in
their work.

Nurses therefore need to question the results of any generic tool
measurements on quality and staffing levels simply on grounds of
validity and reliability. Results should not be accepted meekly as
automatically being 'right' because management 'know what they
are doing'. Constructing a definition of quality is a major task

facing nursing today, for only when we know what quality is will we able to measure it with reliability and validity. We would argue that quality involves dimensions such as compassion, humanity and ethical behaviour: reliance on generic tools will not produce adequate measures of these key aspects of quality nursing care.

This is ongoing work of urgency, but how will this help the nurse in the community or on a hospital ward where generic tools are being used? Can a generic quality tool in its current format help us to value the individual patient and nurse whilst encouraging maximum participation in care? Asking questions about the quality of care and trying to get a measure of this elusive concept, even with the imperfect tools at our disposal today, should help value patients in general, but are the current tools up to the job on an individual basis? Achieving a high score for the ward does not necessarily mean that any individual patient achieves high-quality nursing care or, as many would argue, that the ward is in general delivering high-quality nursing care either.

Producing figures on a ward-by-ward basis does not reflect care received by any individual patient, especially when those figures omit the vital psychosocial dimension of nurse–patient interaction. The criteria set in these tools are, by definition, general and therefore more akin to the mass society of Freire (1985) rather than individuals. As Robinson (1990) has rightly pointed out, these tools produce only coarse-grained data collected in an artificial way; they fall short of the fine-grained situational detail required for a valid assessment of quality.

The generic nature of these tools raises another fundamental issue in terms of liberating nursing practice. The standards set within the tools are not those of the staff on the areas in question but of some outside panel of experts. This is contrary to the notion of empowerment, where clinical staff take responsibility and decisions. It is not very empowering to have standards set by an outside authority and to be told, in the words of Evans and English (1992), that quality is 'compliance to requirements'. This smacks of following orders: nurses do not have to think what constitutes good-quality nursing care for their individual patients; they merely have to comply with requirements. Freire's powerful critique of mass society as an oppressed society following the signposts of others is vividly illustrated by this use of the language of compliance. Nursing must reject such an approach if it is ever to reclaim authority over itself.

If management decide to use a generic tool on a ward, or ward staff themselves decide they wish to take such an initiative, it is important that, whilst recognizing the severe limitations of these tools, nurses should try and get the best results out of them, for what they are worth. This means working hard to get to grips with the issue of reliability and spending the time required to ensure that the observers have been properly trained to minimize the subjective and serious threats to reliability that exist.

There needs to be a careful programme of consultation with ward staff to explain the purpose of the exercise. If staff feel this is a management imposition which is being carried out as part of a cost-cutting exercise, then they are not being valued or empowered in any way. The purpose needs to be clarified – that it is about quality of care. Caution is needed here also, as simply stating that it is about checking and improving the quality of care carries the implicit criticism that care is of low quality, hence the need to check. This again is not valuing staff. The full cooperation of the staff is essential if generic tools are to perform to the best of their ability, which means that staff must be fully involved in what is happening and feel they have a stake in the exercise.

Writers such as Harvey (1987) and Goldstone (1987) have claimed that the use of Monitor is advantageous because it makes nurses think about their practice. This is consistent with our arguments that nurses need to adopt a reflective style of working and offers a potential benefit from the use of such tools. If a Monitor exercise, for example, makes nurses look at how they run a ward and brings about change as a result – achieves praxis – this should be welcomed. However, does the tool, as it sets general mass standards, value the individual clinical nurse and his/her expertise?

In summing up these thoughts it seems that there are a few positive aspects of generic tools: they allow nurses to speak to managers in a language they understand, they may promote reflection upon care, and with sufficient effort invested in training may produce results which might measure some general aspects of care on a macro-ward level.

Set against this are the disadvantages that generic methods fail to capture much of the richness of nursing care; they deny nurses any participation in quality measurement as standards are imposed from above; they are underpinned by a philosophy of compliance; and, crucially, they lack reliability and validity. Generic tools fail many of the tests of empowerment and liberation nursing which we have advocated and their use should only be seen as one imperfect way of measuring just one aspect of quality. Interpretation of findings should be attempted only in the context of a thorough grasp of reliability and validity issues. A great deal of work needs to be done before these approaches can be relied upon to produce valid measures of the quality of nursing care, and as a result, contribute to the empowerment of patients and nurses.

Peer-group methods

This approach to quality differs from the preceding methods on the very important aspect of who is setting the standards, for here staff set their own standards by mutual agreement. It is at once a more empowering approach.

The Royal College of Nursing (RCN) have pioneered work in this field with the dynamic standard setting system (Kitson 1988). The general principle involves groups of clinical staff setting their own standards and consequently monitoring and evaluating their own practice. Standards are seen as a level of performance which is desired and which should be agreed by the group in relation to any particular problem. They are therefore behavioural in nature and in order to measure their achievement it is necessary to establish criteria for success. We therefore come to know standards by their associated criteria. Staff then have to agree measurement techniques and courses of action to achieve the set standard.

An example of a standard might be that the nursing process will be used to facilitate individualized patient-centred care. Criteria that would allow the nurse to know that standard was being achieved might be the presence of up-to-date, written care plans, which had individualized problem and goal statements and nursing interventions clearly identified that related to those goals.

Kemp and Richardson (1990) acknowledge that this approach has much to recommend it, but caution that a great deal of care has to go into making the group work effectively. They suggest a size of between four and six members which should include somebody from outside the immediate ward team, such as a tutor. The group needs to meet frequently (e.g. twice a month) or else momentum will be lost. There needs to be a general discussion concerning values and philosophy, the meanings of quality to different members and the purpose of the whole exercise. It is possible to become bogged down at this stage so too much time should not be spent here. However,

misunderstandings which may arise later due to differing perceptions on such fundamental aspects may be avoided by discussion
early on. Topics to be chosen may be ones that are giving cause for
concern or which members feel are important; a sense of priority is
needed as not everything will be amenable to action in the first
instance.

Consideration must be given to the issues of validity and
reliability. Are the criteria which have been set really measuring
achievement of a standard? To go back to the fundamental question,
is something measuring what it says it is measuring? If we refer to
the example of a standard about use of the nursing process, a
criterion might be that there is a care plan at the foot of every bed.
However, if that care plan is out of date or contains generalized
statements about care that are equally found in many other care
plans, clearly individualized, patient-centred care is not occurring
and the criterion that there will be a care plan at the foot of every bed
is not valid. Reliability must also be tested. Do nurses agree on the
meaning of a criterion so that there is consistency when evaluation
takes place? A criterion such as the presence of patient-centred goals
in the care plan will be unreliable if staff do not agree on what is a
patient-centred goal. Problems such as these require the standard-
setting group to have access to somebody with experience of
research to advise on these crucial issues.

The RCN approach incorporates the classic analysis of Donabedian (1966) who wrote of quality in terms of structure, process and
outcome. Structure refers to factors such as staffing, facilities and
other aspects of the environment; process the actual carrying out of
care; and outcome looks at the results of care. Quality is such a
multifaceted entity that debates about which of these three aspects
offers the best way of measuring it are of little value. No one
measure can capture the complexity of nursing care, as we have
stated already, therefore all three dimensions should be used. The
RCN methodology therefore requires the setting of criteria which
reflect the three dimensions of structure, process and outcome.

An alternative peer-group approach is known as quality circles.
These consist of groups of staff from a common work area meeting
regularly to address problems. A key characteristic is that various
grades and types of staff are involved – anybody who has a
legitimate point of view about a problem in fact. There is no room
for élitism in a quality circle as each member of staff has a valid
point of view. Teamwork and good communication are potential

benefits from this approach, in addition to bringing together a range of perspectives which can help solve a problem. Standards and criteria may also be developed by such an *ad hoc* group. The origin of quality circles is usually credited to Japanese manufacturing industry and they have much in common with the flexible, 'chunking' approach advocated for problem-solving in Chapter 4.

There are certain areas where peer-group quality work is very difficult because of problems associated with getting staff together in one room long enough and often enough to achieve any results. Community staff might be one example, permanent night staff another. There is a peer-group approach which can work however, and that is a research method known as the Delphi technique. It aims to build a consensus amongst staff about key issues, starting from a very open-ended position. The approach is to ask open-ended questions in a questionnaire about whatever the entity is under investigation, then, by analysing the content of responses, picking out key themes. A second-stage questionnaire contains statements prepared from the content analysis and asks staff to rate each statement in order of importance or agreement using, for example, a Likert scale. After analysis a third stage is possible – although it involves sacrificing anonymity – in which all participants are sent a copy of their own responses together with the overall group response and asked how much they agree with the group picture. In this way a consensus can be built from amongst a group of subjects without the need for any formal meeting.

An example of this approach in action has been provided by Hewitt-Sayer and Mayfield (1992), who used the Delphi techniques to obtain agreement amongst night staff about standards of care. They circulated an open-ended questionnaire and from the responses derived 69 factors which staff felt influenced the kind of night a patient might have. On the second questionnaire staff were asked to rate the importance of each factor on a four-point scale. Staff were then informed of the group response and their own response and asked if they wished to alter their views in the light of this feedback. From this exercise it was possible to identify the key factors around which standards and quality work should proceed for night-duty staff.

A significant problem with this work concerns the response rate to the first questionnaire, which was quoted as only 28.6%. To what extent are the views of the staff who responded representative of those who did not? Non-response bias is the name given to this sort of problem in the research literature and studies with response rates of below 40% are usually rejected as being unreliable because of possible bias. If this approach is to be taken to quality, it is essential that a much higher response rate than barely a quarter be achieved if the process of factor identification is to be reliable.

Peer-group quality work is undoubtedly much more empowering as it involves all members of the nursing team and thereby generates a sense of ownership and values the individual nurse. It escapes from the problem of generic quality tools in that standards can be set which are flexible and realistic for the care environment in question. However, they are also relative standards and herein lies a dilemma. A standard which is acceptable on one ward may not be on another. If ward x sets a low standard for pressure care and achieves it 98% of the time, while ward y sets a much higher standard and only achieves it 85% of the time, which is the better ward and which patients are getting the better care?

The peer-group approach to standards suffers from the problem of comparability between clinical areas. One answer might be to set up a trust- or authority-wide committee with the job of equalizing standards between wards or community areas. This still means that it is not possible to compare one trust with the next, for example, and with quality being cited as a key factor in purchasing decisions, this assumes major importance. It is worth noting that what the chief executive of a purchasing authority means by quality may be very different from a clinical nurse.

Setting up trust-level quality committees will involve a great deal of hard work and tact as it may destroy the sense of ownership and empowerment that the peer-group approach brings with it. Girvin (1990) has described with commendable honesty how her health authority got it wrong in this way by trying to have a very top-down, centralized approach to standard-setting. The problems of resentment this caused amongst staff were exacerbated by a lack of any clear and agreed purpose as to why the exercise was to be carried out. The situation was only turned around and got on to the right track after realizing that a bottom-up approach from ward level was needed. Management had to let go of the reins and allow the clinical staff to develop their own standards, following facilitator training with the RCN system.

An obvious problem with the peer-group standard-setting approach is that there might be a great deal of duplication of effort as groups of nurses labour long and hard to write similar standards for similar clinical areas up and down the country. Reinventing the wheel is a wasteful use of scarce professional nursing time.

The RCN has therefore been publishing collections of standards for various clinical areas which staff can adapt for themselves. This seems a sensible approach which still allows staff a sense of ownership and ensures that standards are sensitive to local needs. Knott and Wilkinson (1992) give a good example of adapting the RCN system to their own requirements but conclude with the fatal mistake of asserting, without any evidence to support their claim, that standard-setting has led to higher standards of care. They also make no mention of checking that in the adaptation process whatever reliability and validity the RCN system possesses has not been compromised. Nursing cannot afford to make these mistakes, particularly in print.

In setting standards there is inevitably going to be conflict between what nurses think is desirable and what NHS management can afford and therefore what management thinks is desirable. Mackenzie (1992) poses the telling question that, if finance is so restricted, how can nurses ever set standards which are more than barely adequate? The issue of accountability is raised here because another factor to consider in setting standards is that they should be such that nurses can be held accountable for them.

A case known to one of the authors illustrates the point. A ward team identified the need for raised toilet seats to enhance patient comfort and dignity as part of their quality of care work. Management refused to entertain the idea because the budget was exhausted – there simply was not the money available. When the senior nurse on the ward produced calculations which showed that there would be significant savings from the new seats, management immediately purchased them, despite the 'exhausted budget' (a remarkable recovery!). The nurses felt angry as they perceived this as cost-driven care disguised as quality-driven care.

This example raises some very interesting issues, the prime one of which seems to be that for any quality initiative to succeed, there has to be a dividend which management can identify as saving money. Quality therefore has to be self-financing. In a cash-strapped NHS, this may not be surprising, but perhaps some senior NHS managers and politicians could spare us their hypocritical humbug about quality and be honest – quality improvements must pay for themselves as government is not able or willing to find the extra money otherwise required.

To set standards which are unachievable is disastrous for at least two reasons. First, if nurses fail to achieve these standards, staff morale will plunge as the ward is labelled a failure. Second, if accountability is to mean what it says, i.e. be a valid concept in nursing, then the nurse will be held responsible for ensuring that care of an agreed standard is delivered. If the criteria for standard achievement are not met, the nurse is in serious professional trouble. Lack of resources will be seen at best as a lame excuse showing poor professional judgement by the nursing staff in the first place for setting such unrealistic standards. It would have been far better to set a standard which was realistic for the resources available and argue that, with more resources, higher standards would be possible. Pushing this argument further, if nurses have no control over resources, how can they ever be held accountable for anything? Standard-setting could therefore be a waste of time.

An absolute bottom line in standard-setting might be the UKCC *Code of Professional Conduct*. Many nurses however have a serious credibility problem with this piece of paper, which management seem to ignore at will. It certainly did not help Graham Pink in his battles with management over standards of care.

Peer-group quality assurance by standard-setting has the potential to degenerate into another nursing ritual. It is important that staff stand back and ask why they are wanting to engage in such time-consuming activity. There must be a clear and agreed sense of purpose amongst staff. The danger of not seeing the wood for the trees is real as staff may try to write standards about everything without asking themselves why? Koch (1992) has pointed out the potential for confusion if nurses are not sure why they are writing standards, as this may lead to a great deal of wasted time writing standards which are unnecessary or irrelevant. A plethora of standards may have the effect of fragmenting nursing care and reducing it again to a task-focused exercise.

Setting standards for everything, as Mackenzie (1992) rightly points out, will not produce a blueprint for ideal nursing practice because 'everything' has to be defined. A standard cannot be set for something until we know what that something is. It is far better, writes Mackenzie, to adopt a more realistic approach and avoid trying to set standards for an infinite number of situations and concrete tasks, but rather to set them for principles. If the principles of care are hallmarked by quality, then a crucial step in quality assurance has been taken.

A good example of not seeing the wood for the trees is provided in a paper by Ingram and Woodward (1991), who describe how they set a standard that, to improve pressure care, *every* patient admitted to their elderly care unit would be placed on a ripple mattress. This misses the fundamental principle of individualized patient care and also, on another level, ignores the basic principles of pressure-sore prevention. The effect of this standard is to focus care on to pressure-relieving beds as the means of preventing pressure sores. Alternative methods are excluded as the scope for nursing intervention is foreclosed. The wood in this case contains trees such as 2-hourly turns, early mobilization, enhanced nutrition and hydration, friction-reducing methods such as correct lifting techniques and sheepskins, all of which are excluded by the focus on pressure-relieving beds. There was no way of monitoring if this standard was achieved, other than 'informal checking'. The standard was used as evidence to management, that more pressure-relieving beds were needed, for which the money was not available; consequently the standard was unobtainable. A broader, principle-based approach might have produced a happier outcome.

The authors also report that the introduction of this standard in a top-down fashion was greeted with resentment by staff who interpreted it as a criticism of their pressure care. Standard-setting is doomed to failure if it is seen as a top-down management exercise depending upon coercive methods. This is a cautionary tale of how standard-setting can become ritualistic and counterproductive.

If we return to our themes of empowerment and liberation, peer-group approaches to quality appear to have much to recommend them. Quality circles or standard-setting groups can be run in an empowering way which values the contribution that individual nurses can make, as long as they are bottom-up exercises, based in the clinical areas. They also have the potential to allow the patient's voice to be heard, thereby offering empowerment to the consumer of health care. In setting standards, why not ask the patient's point of view? This can also be incorporated into the Delphi technique, as Hewitt-Sayer and Mayfield (1992) showed. It is possible that patients may have a very different perspective on quality and in Hewitt-Sayer and Mayfield's study, patients picked out some very different quality factors to nursing staff.

The peer-group exercise should lead to reflection upon practice: why are we doing what we are doing and can we do it better? A non-threatening, collaborative atmosphere is essential, however, making the facilitator's role pivotal to the success of the group. Knowledge of research is essential from both a methodological perspective (reliability and validity) and to ensure that realistic standards are set. Very careful scrutiny of criteria to ensure they relate to standards in a valid way is necessary if the RCN approach is to be meaningful. Research into this linkage is needed for the future development of standard-setting.

Standard-setting cannot proceed without proper training of staff to ensure they do not waste time setting standards about the wrong sort of things. As Koch asserts, it is a lamentable state of affairs if, after a huge investment of nursing time and effort, the results are left gathering dust in some long-forgotten cupboard. Standard-setting must relate to the real world in a practical, achievable sense and be something that the staff want to do, rather than having been pressurized into doing by management. Standards relating to a few crucial principles will be more useful and a better utilization of time than trying to write standards about everything. Working with principles requires a shift in thinking away from the concrete to the more conceptual.

Peer-group standard-setting gives power back to nurses as it can be seen to help them regain control over their own destinies, subject to the issue of resources, discussed earlier. Patients can also be brought into the mainstream of care by being involved in peer-group work. It encourages reflection upon practice and facilitates changes in practice by doing. Praxis is therefore a potential consequence of such an exercise and evidence should actively be sought to show that peer-group standard-setting really has improved care. Without that evidence it is difficult to justify the time and effort however.

There are therefore potentially many empowering benefits from this approach. The difficulties that have been outlined in this section should not be glossed over, however, and many of the problems raised under the preceding, generic section are relevant also. Staff must want to become involved in this work, have a clear sense of purpose and an understanding of the research process if the time is to be spent constructively. There are many ways of using peer groups to develop quality: nurses should avoid the trap of thinking that there is such a thing as the single right method and always remember that there is more to quality than numbers. Evaluation of quality should contain more than percentages and never be based upon one dimension, such as process; it is far too complex for that. A final consideration should be that standards are always relative and depend upon an underlying philosophy. Nurses should not therefore be surprised if their standards differ from colleagues and other professional groups within the health-care arena.

Patient satisfaction measures

The issue of consumer-led quality measurement leads into patient satisfaction ratings. Providers of health care such as NHS trusts, anxious to attract business, are one obvious group to whom patient satisfaction ratings of quality are very attractive. The apparent simplicity of collecting the data compared to the complex and time-consuming administration of generic tools or peer-group methodologies makes patient satisfaction ratings appealing to management. Nurses wishing to understand the nature of the patient's experiences are also attracted to this approach, but are realizing that questionnaires, although apparently quick and simple, are very limited in the information they can gather. It is likely that evaluations of patient satisfaction will be increasingly used in a market-oriented NHS.

Patient satisfaction ratings have a common-sense appeal about them as they have face validity, i.e. 'on the face of it' asking patients to assess the quality of their care seems an obvious step. It appears to involve patients in care and therefore has potential for patient empowerment, providing that staff listen to the patients' comments and act accordingly. This rider is crucial, otherwise there is no point if staff become defensive and dismiss any critical comments. Many patients are not able to participate in this approach to quality assurance, however, by virtue of intellectual impairment or immaturity.

The issues of reliability and validity must be addressed in some depth. Patient satisfaction surveys have been shown to suffer from a lack of discriminatory ability; they all seem to show high degrees of patient satisfaction whatever area they are used in (Bond and Thomas, 1992). If they cannot discriminate between good and less good care, can they be said to be reliable? By analogy, bathroom scales cannot distinguish weights that are a few grams apart and therefore cannot be considered a reliable measuring tool for weighing cooking ingredients. There is a view also that a patient response will tend to be biased towards a favourable rating as the patient may feel obliged to say positive things about care or have nothing with which to compare the care given. Reliability is therefore threatened by bias.

The validity of self-rated questionnaires in use with patients is also open to question. Walsh (1991) highlights the situation of a ward operating on a self-care philosophy such as that inherent in Dorothea Orem's approach to nursing. Some patients may not be happy with being required to do things for themselves, feeling that the nursing staff should do more for them; the result might be a negative rating of care that the nursing staff felt was of a high order because of its emphasis on self-care and rehabilitation. Care is a form of communication and social psychologists are well aware that communication given may be interpreted very differently by the person receiving it. The same applies to care – what appears good nursing care to the nurse may not be perceived as such by the patient. This point is underlined by Yorke (1992) who points out that the customer is not always right in assessing quality. To what extent therefore is the patient's satisfaction rating measuring the quality of care given?

Bond and Thomas (1992) hypothesize that a move towards more individualized, patient-centred care may paradoxically lead to an increase in *expressed* patient dissatisfaction simply because patients feel more able to express their own views and complain than they could under a more authoritarian, task-focused regime. A patient satisfaction rating might be less than good or there may be more complaints logged about care, although paradoxically the care would be rated as having improved according to conventional nursing wisdom. These authors are very critical of the lack of consistency in the way patient satisfaction data has been gathered in the past, particularly in studies which claim to support the introduction of primary nursing by assessing patient satisfaction. This issue will be explored further in Chapter 7.

The concept of satisfaction is as subjective as quality itself; consequently it is a dangerous step to state that whatever the patient understands by this term reflects accurately the quality of care given. There are many things that can affect satisfaction besides the actual quality of care. Fitzpatrick (1990) has expressed concern about the lack of investigation into the validity and meaning of the common-sense concept of satisfaction. Because it is a common-sense notion, it has lacked definition and may therefore mean different things to different people, which of course undermines the reliability of the concept.

If patient satisfaction is to be used as a measure of quality, French (1981) has shown that interviews with patients tend to give more reliable information than questionnaires. However, Fitzpatrick (1984) demonstrated that the extent to which the interviewer is identified with the service influences the answers that patients give.

Obtaining the consumer's view of the service offered is therefore an attractive quality-assurance tool, but fraught with problems concerning reliability and validity. In order to use patient satisfaction measures as a means of assessing quality, Bond and Thomas urge the need to define exactly what is meant by patient satisfaction and then link questions with specific aspects of nursing care rather than generalities.

Questionnaires are by nature superficial and therefore an interview approach may obtain more meaningful information, especially if the notion of 'satisfaction' were set aside in designing the interview schedule. The difficulty of defining patient satisfaction and the validity of the concept suggest a better approach might be to explore other areas in the interview which can link to quality. Examples might be pain, comfort, communication, anxiety, feeling valued. Obtaining the patient's views about a range of topics such as these might say a great deal more about the quality of care being *received* than ticking a few boxes rating 'satisfaction'. The word 'received' is crucial for this, the patient's view, and this may be different from the nursing staff's perception, which is of care being administered.

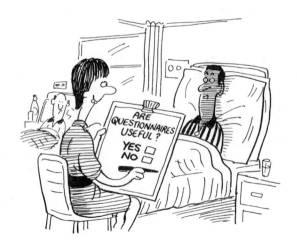

When this brief discussion of patient satisfaction ratings is considered in the light of its liberating potential for nursing, it appears at first glance very promising. Asking the patient's views is potentially very empowering for the patient, providing this is done in such a way that the patient feels able to be honest in answering the questions and the nursing staff are prepared to reflect and act upon the answers. Benner's discussion (1984) of critical incidents and their effect upon nursing links into this concept, for patient feedback is an excellent source of learning for the nurse. We must listen to patients for, in the process, we learn much about ourselves.

It is the place of a research text to explore all the various issues such as bias, sampling, clarity of phrasing questions, threats to validity and reliability. Suffice it to say that a patient satisfaction measure is a serious research undertaking and requires knowledge of survey research techniques before it can be undertaken in such a way as to produce meaningful data. These issues need to be addressed before embarking on such an exercise. The laudable goals of empowerment and quality care demand and deserve a thorough approach. There are no easy short cuts.

The contribution of quality assurance to nursing empowerment

The three views of quality assurance that have been presented so far offer varying degrees of potential benefit to patient care, but are each surrounded by problems. Nursing has taken quality seriously in the UK and should continue to do so; however, in common with other aspects of nursing, we should not accept uncritically what is urged upon us. There are many blind alleyways in the quality assurance maze and we should use our basic nursing principles of empowerment and liberation as signposts to help us find our way rather than accept unquestioningly the directions of the first person we encounter with a clipboard under the arm.

Total quality management (TQM) is concerned with ensuring that quality is not the subject of sporadic initiatives and task forces, but rather pervades every pore of an organization. Everybody should be involved in quality, according to Mudie (1991). TQM is about encouraging, recognizing and valuing the contribution that all staff can make, but this requires a change of strategy because at present the NHS is sadly not like that. She recommends a normative–educative approach to such a change (see p. 67), urging managers to avoid a coercive 'big brother' style.

Nursing should be comfortable with the notion of TQM, especially when, according to Muller and Funnell (1991) it can lead to benefits such as greater use of team work, eliminating wasteful and unproductive activities, greater identification with the customer and a greater emphasis on prevention of problems. These authors were actually writing in an industrial context and a great deal of what is written about quality is transferrable across contexts – though not all.

It is possible to agree strongly with their view that quality demands the involvement of all staff as valued participants; it is about people, not procedures. The danger exists that in setting standards we become so obsessed with the procedures of standard-setting that we forget why we are doing it – for the benefit of people – and who is doing it – other people called nurses. The aim should be to release creativity and innovation rather than the imposition of procedures which enforce conformity of standards. That way lies the re-creation of the procedure manual and the 'we've always done it this way' mentality, reinforced by 'because it's a standard and we must comply with requirements'. Shelley (1992) has warned of cumbersome quality manuals with standards for everything choking individualized nursing care. The way forwards, as we have argued, is to write standards about principles, allowing nurses flexibility to develop practice.

Nursing will have lost its soul if compliance with requirements is the best definition we can offer of quality nursing care, yet this is a definition encountered in industry which is being transmitted into health care by messiahs who would lead us to the promised land of the market place. Quality is much more than the cost of doing things wrong – another myopic definition borrowed from industry and offered by Evans and English (1992). Such a definition is as accurate as describing a great classical concerto as a collection of notes. As we have noted, not everything in the industrial management textbooks translates into nursing: nursing is too complex for that.

There is another notion of quality, drawn from education, which sees it as transforming the consumer (Barnett, 1992, Yorke, 1992) and adding value to that person by the educational process. By analogy, to what extent does health care result in a transformation of the patient? Is the individual more independent, in less pain, better able to cope? If we could show that care has transformed patients in a materially beneficial way, then we could really argue for quality. This requires shifting the emphasis away from process and structure, the main preoccupations of much of the work discussed in this chapter, towards outcomes. What can the patient do now that s/he could not do without nursing intervention? This seems a very pertinent question to ask if we wish to demonstrate the quality and value of nursing care, especially in a results-oriented, market-driven health-care system, such as is now developing in the UK.

To measure the transforming nature of care requires both objective and subjective measurement. If a thorough patient assessment has been carried out initially, it should be possible to demonstrate improvements which may be quantified such as distance walked unaided, reduction in numbers of incontinence episodes per day or knowledge about self-medication. Subjective information concerning patients' moods, feelings about themselves, pain or anxiety levels should also be collected to demonstrate change or transformation. Interviews are more appropriate than a questionnaire approach in gathering this sort of information as they allow the patient's full realm of experience to be explored.

This approach to quality assurance puts the patient at the centre of the exercise in a way that process and structure measures do not because they tend to focus on the nurse's perspective. Patient empowerment demands that the patient be the focal point of quality assurance. An obvious point that might be raised is that such an approach makes it impossible to distinguish how much of the patient's improvement is attributable to nursing care and how much to other professional groups. From the patient's perspective, does it matter? Are we being parochial in trying to claim $x\%$ of the improvement in patient A as being down to nursing only? If we do more than pay lip service to multidisciplinary teamwork and actually make it reality, then should the argument be that the health-care team produced this amount of change for the better?

Nurses might feel worried about the loss of nursing as a distinctive entity within this approach. The antinursing, antiprofessional bias of many senior managers in the NHS today makes this totally reasonable. One approach might be initially to carry out research which does focus in a narrow sense on the value of nursing before moving on to this more integrated approach. Perhaps it will be a sign of real nursing maturity and empowerment when we feel confident in taking our place within such a multidisciplinary team and concentrate on measuring the improvement in the quality of the patient's life which results from a *team* approach to care.

The need for collaboration with other professional groups in measuring quality has been stressed by the General Secretary of the RCN, Christine Hancock (1991), along with the development of a common vocabulary of terms to avoid confusion over different meanings. Hancock also went on to criticize the failure of health professionals to address issues of outcomes in quality measurement. We would support this change of emphasis: outcome must have a much higher priority in quality measurement, although not completely at the expense of structure and process. Quality is so complex that it needs measuring from every possible angle if we are to get an accurate picture, including the effect of the care provided in transforming the quality of life of the patient.

In conclusion, therefore, we can see that the quality of nursing care is an issue that is every nurse's business. If we do not set the agenda and pursue methods and standards which we think as a profession are appropriate, we will find others imposing their own standards with little regard for nursing or for the patient, both of whom will be losers. Empowerment and liberation can be greatly facilitated by a strong nursing quality drive which incorporates patient perspectives.

Such development needs to acknowledge that there are many different aspects to quality and that there is no single, simple measure of such an elusive and complex entity. Nurses undertaking quality assurance work must want to do it for themselves, understand why they are doing it, and be aware that what they are undertaking is research and therefore requires certain skills, particularly in relation to observation and measurement. An alternative approach to quality has been suggested to complement the existing mainstream methods in which it should be understood in terms of transformation. What difference did health care make to the patient's life? The patient's point of view should be pivotal in this approach and it should be obtained by other techniques than just ticking boxes on questionnaires.

A simplistic, management-driven, one-track approach to quality may well lead to another generation of nursing rituals and care being standardized to death. Those who would argue that there is only one way to assess quality, and it happens to be their way, should be ignored as likely members of the UFM (Union of False Messiahs).

References

Allen M (1991) When the GM invites the porter to lunch. *Nursing* 1991 **4**: 2.
Balogh R (1992) Audits of nursing care in Britain; a review and a critique of approaches to validating them. *International Journal of Nursing Studies* **29**: 119–133.
Barnett D, Wainwright P (1987) Between two stools. *Senior Nurse* **6**: 40–42.
Barnett R (1992) *Improving Higher Education*. Milton Keynes, Society for Research into Higher Education and OU Press.
Benner P (1984) *From Novice to Expert*. Menlo Park, CA, Addison-Wesley.
Bond S, Thomas L (1992) Measuring patients' satisfaction with nursing care. *Journal of Advanced Nursing* **17**: 52–63.
Department of Health (1992) *Health of the Nation*. London, Department of Health.
Donabedian A (1966) Evaluating the quality of nursing care. *Millbank Memorial Fund Quarterly* **2**: 166–206.
Evans K, English G (1992) Introducing total quality management. *Nursing Standard* **6**: 27, 32–35.
Everett B, Hay D (1992) *Talking About Statistics*. London, Edward Arnold.
Fitzpatrick R (1984) Satisfaction with health care. In: Fitzpatrick R (ed) *The Experience of Illness*. London, Tavistock.
Fitzpatrick R (1990) Measurement of patient satisfaction. In: Hopkins A, Costain D (eds) *Measuring the Outcomes of Medical Care*. London, Royal College of Physicians.
Freire P (1985) *The Politics of Education; Culture, Power and Liberation*. New York, Macmillan.
French K (1981) Methodological considerations in hospital opinion surveys. *International Journal of Nursing Studies* **18**: 7–32.
Gault A (1982) The Aberdeen formula as an illustration of the difficulty of determining nursing requirements. *International Journal of Nursing Studies* **19**: 61–77.
Girvin J (1990) Setting standards; uphill work. *Nursing Standard* **4**: 44, 34–35.
Goldstone L (1987) Monitor. In: Pearson A (ed) *Nursing Quality Measurement*. Chichester, John Wiley.
Hancock C (1991) Multi-disciplinary clinical audit. *Nursing Standard* **5**: 18, 37.
Harvey G (1987) Compiling a directory. *Nursing Times* **83**: 46, 49–50.
Hewitt-Sayer W, Mayfield S (1992) Night-watch. *Nursing Times* **88**: 15, 32–35.
Ingram C, Woodward M (1991) Choosing the right tools for the job. *Professional Nurse* November, 110-116.
Kemp N, Richardson E (1990) *Quality Assurance in Nursing Practice*. Oxford, Butterworth-Heinemann.
Kitson A (1988) *Nursing Quality Assurance–Dynamic Standard Setting System*. London, RCN Standards of Care Project.
Knott P, Wilkinson E (1992) A measure of care. *Nursing Times* **88**: 16, 28–30.
Koch T (1992) A review of nursing quality assurance. *Journal of Advanced Nursing* **17**: 785–794.
Mackenzie J (1992) Dilemmas in setting quality standards. *Nursing Standard* **6**: 29, 37–39.
Markham G (1988) Dividing the day. *Nursing Times* **84**: 32, 29–30.

Mudie S (1991) TQM: Everyone's business. *Nursing* **4**: 39, 26–28.

Muller D, Funnell P (1991) *Delivering Quality in Vocational Education.* London, Kagan Page.

Norman I, Redfern S, Tomalin D, Oliver S (1992) Applying triangulation to the assessment of the quality of nursing. *Nursing Times* **88**: 8, 43–46.

Polit D, Hungler B (1987) *Nursing Research; Principles and Methods.* Philadelphia, Lippincott.

Robinson D (1990) Qualitative analysis of care. *Senior Nurse* **10**: 21–25.

Shelley H (1992) Mission impossible? *Nursing Times* **88**: 16, 37.

Tomalin D, Redfern S, Norman I (1992) Monitor and senior monitor: problems of administration and some proposed solutions. *Journal of Advanced Nursing* **17**: 72–82.

UKCC (1992) *Code of Professional Conduct.* London, UKCC.

Walsh M (1991) *Nursing Models in Clinical Practice; The Way Forward.* London, Baillière Tindall.

Yorke (1992) Quality in higher education: a conceptualisation and some observations on the implementation of a sector quality system. *Journal of Further and Higher Education* **16**: 90–104.

7 Primary nursing

Introduction

The arrival of primary nursing from the USA might be seen as one of the single most important developments in UK nursing in the last couple of decades. There is now a vast volume of nursing literature advocating the cause of primary nursing whilst, in 1992, the Prime Minister himself appeared to give it the official seal of approval by announcing his named nurse initiative. But there are questions and doubts – there is the danger that nursing is being swept away by a tide of enthusiasm and not using its critical faculties adequately. There are voices in the wilderness raising difficult issues and arguing that the advocates of primary nursing have failed to construct a research-based case for their cause. This latter point is crucial, for in the absence of research evidence supporting such a major change in the way nursing is delivered, it is hard to see how implementation of primary nursing may proceed except as another ritual.

If the nurse practitioner concept discussed in Chapter 8 is to develop and grow in the future, nursing needs to establish that as a profession it can be held accountable for its actions and display a reasonable degree of autonomy. The primary nurse must also demonstrate these qualities as s/he manages a patient caseload. The primary nurse role may therefore be thought of as a precursor to the nurse practitioner for it is hard to see a nurse who could not take on a primary nurse role in a hospital ward progressing to the even more autonomous role of nurse practitioner. The importance of primary nursing is therefore twofold – it represents a major nursing development in its own right, and is an essential precursor to an even bigger initiative, the nurse practitioner.

In this chapter we shall examine what is meant by primary nursing, how the ideal fits with the notions of liberation nursing we have discussed earlier, and then look at the reality of practice. If the concept of primary nursing is flawed or too narrow as presently understood, there are huge implications for the future credibility of nursing. A hasty and ill-thought-out campaign of implementation that misfired would be a blow from which nursing may take decades to recover.

What is primary nursing?

Most nurses have a working definition that involves the notion of an individual nurse taking responsibility for a group of patients on a 24-hour basis. This nurse is the primary nurse and is responsible for admitting and discharging the patient, planning all care in between. A similar definition applies in community settings; however, most of the research has focused on the hospital environment. When the nurse is off duty, associate nurses carry on the care according to the care plan. A primary nurse for one group of patients may also be an associate nurse for others. This simplified description covers the basic elements of Manthey's original description (1980) which concentrated on how care is organized.

This says little however about what the nature of that care should be. A great deal more has been written extending the concept of primary nursing into a much wider field concerning the nature of care itself. This has sown the seeds of confusion and doubt as what one person understands by primary nursing may not be the same as another. Macdonald (1988) has shown how a range of abstract concepts such as autonomy, accountability, comprehensiveness and co-ordination have been added to the original organizational definition along with other concepts such as advocacy, assertiveness, authority, collaboration, continuity and commitment. As Macdonald points out, the ever-widening definitions have become so all-encompassing that they have moved on from a definition of a method of organizing care to a new philosophy of care and on to positively Utopian visions of nursing! The danger with such ever-widening definitions is that they become useless and the original concept gets lost in the swirling clouds of idealism.

Has primary nursing now come to mean everything that we believe to be good in nursing? There is nothing wrong in that, except that such a definition is different from the original and has been arrived at via various other definitions on the way. Now, for purposes of implementation, research and evaluation, which definition are we working with? Unless everybody means the same thing by a definition of primary nursing, researching the notion of primary nursing will be a waste of time as different people will be looking at different things but calling them the same name, a recipe for confusion! The same comment applies to implementation: different nurses may be trying to implement different things, all under the broad heading of primary nursing.

Further, any concept which is to be evaluated has to be researchable. In other words it has to be of a manageable size that can be recognized and measured (operationalized, to use research jargon). 'Everything that is good in nursing' cannot be operationalized; it is just too loose a definition to be researched in any practical way. Philosophies do not work well as independent variables in the research process.

This problem was acknowledged by Bond *et al.* (1991) in their study which compared two elderly care wards, one of which was using a team nursing system and the other had converted to primary nursing. These researchers drew up a series of clearly defined organizational criteria for primary nursing which involved staff accepting 24-hour responsibility for a group of patients during their entire stay in hospital and a duty rota which was organized to facilitate this. However, the authors felt that they had to investigate the styles of patient care before they could be satisfied that primary nursing was indeed being practised on the 'experimental' ward. Organization of staff was insufficient to define primary nursing; the style of care was considered equally important. Primary nursing was seen as being about process as well as structure.

The features of care on the experimental ward which the researchers felt showed it practised primary nursing included a large degree of patient involvement in care-planning, continuity of care and good communication through all levels of staffing. As a style of nursing this meets many of the desirable criteria that we outlined in Chapter 5; however, there is nothing in many definitions of primary nursing to cover these areas, Bond *et al.* are working with their own definition and subjectively interpreting what they saw as primary nursing.

The issue is that nurses have set up the organizational model of primary nursing and then extrapolated on into desirable outcomes that should flow from such a method of delivering care, incorporating these into the definition. As a result, the definition has grown and expanded subjectively over the years. As Macdonald argues (1988), it is difficult to differentiate between the aims of primary nursing (what nurses think it should achieve) and the claims made on its behalf (what it has done and as a consequence, what it is, for the former shapes the definition of the latter). Increased professionalization, more staff/patient satisfaction, improved quality of care, rehumanizing hospitals, improved quality of care, clinical autonomy and improving the status of nursing are just some of the aims and claims listed by Macdonald from the literature. But are these characteristics of primary nursing which will help us recognize it when we see it, or are they hoped-for gains that will arise out of the implementation of an organizational system built around 24-hour patient responsibility?

If the former, then the definition has been radically expanded for if a ward cannot demonstrate these sort of characteristics, it cannot be said to be practising primary nursing, however it may organize its patient allocation and shift systems.

The fundamental difficulty that has to be resolved before any attempt can be made to evaluate research looking at primary nursing is the question, what definition of primary nursing were the researchers working with?

A significant attempt to resolve this problem was made by Mead (1991) who utilized a panel of 28 experts in the fields of nursing practice, education and management to try and arrive at a valid definition of primary nursing which could be used as a yardstick to measure implementation. Mead was very aware of the lack of a workable definition as primary nursing has come to mean all things to all nurses, hence her study. As she stated, it is more than allocating patients to nurses: concepts such as devolved decision-making, nurse–patient partnership in care-planning, continuity of care and patient-centred nursing are just some of the concepts that may be involved.

Mead asked a series of six open-ended questions, such as: 'If you went on a ward, how would you know primary nursing was taking place?' and collated the replies from each of her 28 experts. Questions such as these exclude community care and other areas such as theatres and accident and emergency. Grouping the responses she then recirculated each member of her panel of 28 experts with statements drawn from all respondents in the initial trawl and asked them to rate the statements according to how much they agreed with them.

The most interesting finding was the lack of agreement on the fundamental question in the preceding paragraph. Many of the statements that were made by individuals, when circulated to the rest of the group, produced polarized responses either strongly agreeing or disagreeing. In other words, this group of 28 experts could not agree upon the sort of things that would indicate that primary nursing was taking place on any ward they walked on to. Another finding amongst the 28 experts was a group of 10 clinicians for whom over 90% of ratings were strongly yes to whatever statement was made about primary nursing. Mead interprets this as either indicating that these nurses have very poor powers of discrimination, or that for them, primary nursing has become a euphemism for all that is good in nursing.

A lack of discriminatory powers or critical faculties amongst clinical experts in the field of primary nursing raises serious doubts when taken in conjunction with our warning to beware false messiahs. Such individuals could very easily be taken in by visions of the promised land and other nurses in their turn may follow. Conversely, if primary nursing has come to mean good nursing, the philosophy of care and the organizational principles for the delivery of care have become entangled. If primary nursing can be shown to produce a higher quality of care, what is it that has produced the result? Is it the different method of organizing care or is it a new philosophy of what care should be, or both? The question is impossible to answer without disentangling the elements of what people mean by primary nursing.

Mead's final analysis of the response produced the following list of characteristics which identify primary nursing:

- Accountability, authority and responsibility for patient caseload.
- Care centred around individual patient needs.
- Case load attachment from admission to discharge.
- Continuity of care.
- Primary nurse is care-giver.
- Evidence of a value system or ward philosophy.
- Decentralized decision-making.
- Care plans and communication pathways showing the primary nurse as the principal organizer of care.
- Changes in ward organization and skill mix.
- Patient/relative involvement and choice in care.
- Evidence of role changes for nurses involved.
- Development of collegiate relationships.
- Patients know their primary nurse.
- Visual evidence of a system.

From this list it is clear that there is a great deal more to primary nursing than the initial simple definition on p. 126. This list also shows the Prime Minister's apparent conversion to the cause with his named nurse initiative (1992) to be what it was, a cheap electoral gimmick. The notion that one named nurse is responsible for a patient's entire care is but a scrap of canvas compared to the portrait of primary nursing painted by Mead's analysis. Many people think the named nurse initiative is primary nursing. It is not, but this point only underlines the difficulties caused by having so many different definitions of primary nursing.

In summary, primary nursing means different things to different people. It can mean one nurse being responsible for all nursing care received by patients on his/her patch. The ward sister or district nurse/health visitor has always filled that definition and could legitimately be called a named nurse already. Alternatively it can mean a way of organizing care and shift patterns or it can move on to encompass a radical range of points of view about the nature of the relationships between nurses and patients or other nurses or even the very philosophy of care itself. This wide range of meanings must be borne in mind in the rest of this chapter. Any nurse wishing to implement primary nursing therefore needs to think carefully about what is meant by primary nursing and to discuss carefully with colleagues the planned changes, in order to ensure that everybody is working towards the same goal.

An important cautionary note has to be made however. Too many nurses feel under pressure to adopt primary nursing as the only professional way to nurse. This is unfortunate and is particularly unhelpful in terms of developing quality services. The most professional nurses are those who explore a new idea and accept, reject or adapt it according to its relevance to their service requirements. The following discussion will explore these points further.

Primary nursing and the liberation of nursing

Chapter 5 summarized some key aspects of a liberated approach to nursing practice which should now be measured up against Mead's characteristics of primary nursing. The central tenets of liberty include valuing the individual (patient or nurse) and the freedoms of choice and speech. These are fundamental components of the broad picture painted by Mead.

If a nurse is not valued as an individual and given the liberty and authority to choose the nursing care which s/he feels appropriate, then primary nursing cannot work. This simple statement is at odds with the hierarchical traditions of nursing and also the current NHS management's obsession with secrecy and gagging clauses. The implications of such autonomy are profound and need to be carefully explored in the light of primary nursing.

Where authority leads, accountability follows, as night follows day. Yet leading nurses such as Salvage (1985) have argued that it is unfair to hold nurses accountable for the care they deliver as they do not have the authority within the health-care system to ensure adequate staffing and resource levels and will always come into conflict with the medical profession if they try and become too autonomous. Bowers (1989) took issue with this assertion by stating that it leads to the conclusion that nurses are not responsible for anything and he went on to state that nurses are masters (sic) of the art of shifting responsibility on to other professional groups or passing the buck on up the hierarchical ladder.

This analysis is reminiscent of Seligman's ideas of learned helplessness and suggests a striking analogy. Seligman's work began in the realms of experimental psychology (Seligman, 1975) and has now been developed into a model to explain some aspects of adult depressive behaviour (Peterson and Seligman, 1984). The basic idea is that if people believe that their actions make no difference to outcomes, be they pleasurable or unpleasant, then they learn to become helpless, believing there is nothing that can be done. The theory proposes that this belief is associated with a tendency to explain events by attributing them predominantly to internal, stable and global causes. If individuals see the cause for something going wrong as themselves (internal), unlikely to change (stable) and affecting a wide range of things (global) then this works with their belief that nothing they can do will change things to produce depression. Hewstone and Antaki (1988) have pointed out that there is considerable correlational support for this explanation of some forms of depression.

If nursing is considered by analogy, then nursing's subordinate role suggests that we too may have learned to be helpless. We shrug our shoulders and say we have no power and therefore no authority and so cannot be held accountable. In Chapter 1 potential explanations were discussed for nursing's apparent lack of power; many of these reasons lie within nursing (internal). The forces at work have a long history (stable) and affect many other aspects of nurses' lives and health care (global). The necessary conditions for learned helplessness and depression exist on a collective basis for nursing as a whole.

The validity of applying to the collective psyche of nursing a theory that seeks to explain helpless, apathetic behaviour and depression in an individual is admittedly open to challenge. However, the analogy is striking. We have already seen that nurses display many of the characteristics which Freire (1985) has described as being typical of oppressed groups while the ideas of Schon (1983) suggest that nursing, by virtue of its lack of major profession status and perceived serious science base, will always play second fiddle to medicine and management. Nursing has therefore a major credibility problem when it comes to exercising the authority that primary nursing demands. If primary nursing is to be implemented on a wide scale, rather than in a few centres of excellence, the fundamental problem of power and authority that Salvage raised has to be resolved.

If the liberating approach to nursing that is advocated in this book is to be followed and/or if nurses wish to practise primary nursing in its widest sense, then they will have to work to seize the power and authority they require to exercise the autonomy of practice that is needed. The organizational aspects of primary nursing can be made to work without giving nurses any more authority or power, but primary nursing in its philosophical entirety can only be implemented by nurses acquiring real power. Therein lies a danger, for nurses may think that because the organizational trappings of primary nursing are present, they have acquired the power and authority that goes with true autonomy of practice. In this way the named nurse initiative may be a sham which leads nursing into a delusional state that is positively harmful in the long run.

Empowerment, one of the key characteristics of liberated nursing, involves getting rid of hierarchies while groups of staff work together to share decision-making with each other and with the patient. If the primary nurse is the key planner and giver of care, then the traditional nursing hierarchy of staff nurse, sister, manager no longer applies. The vertical hierarchy has been flattened as the ward now has a small group of staff nurses, each equally autonomous and with the same amount of authority, presumably delegated from the ward sister.

McMahon (1990) was able to show significant differences in power distribution in a study comparing two primary nursing wards with a team nursing and a traditionally organized ward. He used a mixture of qualitative and quantitative methods to compare the way the staff worked and to examine the collegial relationships that existed on the differing wards. His observational work indicated that the team nursing ward exhibited a definite hierarchy of power whilst on the traditionally run ward the sister was very much in charge and fixed routines were the norm. On one primary nursing ward he observed a complete absence of anyone in charge as each primary nurse worked independently and had little interaction with other primary nurses, whilst on the other ward the sister had a more influential role and was subtly checking up on the performance of staff nurses who were primary nurses.

McMahon operationalized (turned into a measurable concept) collegiality by adapting a questionnaire that had been devised for use in an American study of nurse educators (Beyer, 1981). Collegiality is understood as the extent to which staff collaborate together in working towards problem solution. The study was piloted but issues of validity or reliability are not addressed. The researcher in his paper therefore does not demonstrate that his questionnaire is measuring what he says it is measuring (collegiality) or that it is doing so accurately, although he asserts this is the case as a result of his adaptation process. This raises the question how can we be sure that what was appropriate for American nurse educators is appropriate for British staff nurses in the NHS? Despite this problem, the results showed that nurses on the primary nursing wards felt their communication with colleagues was significantly more collaborative than on the other two wards. It is worth comparing this staff perception with the lack of interaction between nurses observed on one of the primary nursing wards.

Increased collegiality is consistent with the argument we have advanced for liberating nursing by empowering nurses and suggests that primary nursing has a key role to play. The question remains though, to what extent is this observation due to primary nursing, or has primary nursing been successfully adopted on these wards because a tendency towards collaborative working with minimal hierarchy existed already?

The removal of the vertical hierarchy is welcomed, but empowerment also means sharing decision-making. Staff nurses should therefore discuss care with patients and relatives and also within the staff group. It would be very shortsighted if a primary staff nurse thought that s/he had all the answers and did not discuss patient care with others, such as the enrolled nurse or nursing auxiliary. The primary nurse who was not prepared to share with other (junior) staff in this way is not acting in an empowered way and could be accused of re-creating the old hierarchies on a smaller scale.

Thomas (1992) showed in a study of the way nursing auxiliaries and staff nurses saw their work that there was little difference between the two groups. When primary, team and functional nursing wards were compared, within each type of ward there was no difference in work perception between the two grades of staff and crucially, within the primary nursing wards, nursing auxiliaries used far more initiative and were much more involved than on any of the other wards. Bond *et al.* (1991) have reported similar findings from their studies of primary nursing at work. Thomas (1992) and Bond *et al.* (1991) suggest that within a primary nursing framework, nursing auxiliaries will be able to do far more than follow orders and will be empowered themselves. Thomas concluded that there was a culture within wards, be they primary nursing or any other type, which transcended grade and further that her study argued against the notion of classifying work such that nursing is given only by individuals holding a statutory qualification. She felt that ward culture and philosophy rather than the method of organizing care influenced the perceptions of staff.

If Thomas is correct there are two interesting implications. First, that primary nursing will only work in the fullest sense of the word if the ward philosophy and approach to care are right to start off with. It cannot be imposed upon a ward unless the staff have the commitment to patient-centred care, delegation of authority away from the ward sister and all the other aspects listed by Mead on p. 129. Primary nursing in a way is just codifying good practice. Unless these characteristics exist, or at least there is a predisposition to experiment in this direction, then nurses' names can join consultants above the bed and nurses can call themselves primary and associate nurses, but despite all the organizational trappings, nothing will have changed and primary nursing will not be at work as a philosophy of care. A second implication is that registered nurses must be prepared to accept unqualified staff as worthwhile partners in the delivery of care who have a valid point of view and not re-create the old ward autocracy and hierarchy on a smaller scale.

If getting rid of hierarchies will help liberate nursing, then primary nursing is a very attractive proposition. There are several key issues which need to be thought through, however, particularly surrounding the role of the ward sister/charge nurse. At present the sister is held accountable for the delivery of care to all patients on the ward and is also managerially responsible for staffing and a great deal besides. If clinical responsibility is delegated to primary nurses, what is left for the sister? Do wards need sisters any more if clinical responsibility for patients is taken by primary nurses? Could a member of the clerical staff replace the sister as ward administrator?

There is little in the literature to answer these questions. McCormack's study of primary nursing at work on a surgical ward (McCormack, 1992) showed that staff experienced considerable difficulty in reconciling being in charge of the ward and being a primary nurse. He commented that however much internally nurses may work as a team with clinical responsibility shared, externally, other staff (and the system) still need to identify a person in charge. He also found that internally, whilst recognizing the difficulties this clash caused, nurses themselves still wanted a person in charge of the ward. McCormack also reported that staff felt the primary nurse role was very stressful: this tension between roles can only exacerbate this stress.

This requirement that a single person be identified as in charge and therefore responsible for everything that happens on the ward is more of a problem for hospital staff than in the community. It is also, according to Bowers (1989), ironically a product of a managerial ethos that has contributed to the rise of primary nursing on the NHS agenda in the last few years. Bowers argues that the introduction of general management in the early 1980s after the Griffith enquiry was instrumental in replacing collectivist decision-making with individual responsibility, passed on down a chain of command from regional general manager through districts and units. The managerial ethos therefore required an individual who was taking responsibility for what happened under (usually) him. This fits exactly with primary nursing, which helps explain why managers found the concept appealing as it makes it easy to point the finger at an individual nurse and say 'It's your fault' when things go wrong.

It is interesting to compare sociological trends with nursing developments since 1945. The immediate post-war years were a time when great emphasis was placed on getting the work done; many women had spent years working on production lines in the munitions industries and nursing care in the 1950s and 1960s resembled this approach when functional or task-centred care was at its peak. The late 1960s and 1970s saw the rise of collectivism and cooperatives; nursing moved to the team nursing approach. Then the 1980s saw individualism and New Right ideologies as personified by figures such as Thatcher and Reagan in the ascendency. Nursing moved towards primary nursing, making the individual nurse responsible for all that happened to his/her patients. If nursing trends are indeed shadowing broader social movements, it is intriguing to try and speculate how the society of the early 1990s may influence nursing in the future.

Returning to the present and looking at a primary nursing ward we see a paradox, for if the primary nurse claims autonomy and accountability as justification for her care, and the sister disagrees with the care given, how should the sister/charge nurse act? If s/he tries to interfere in what the primary nurse is doing then primary nursing is no longer being practised according to the purists, but the sister/charge nurse is also being held managerially accountable by higher authority for all that happens on the ward, therefore to do nothing puts him/her in danger of dismissal for negligence. It is difficult to see how the sister/charge nurse can reconcile managerial responsibility with the clinical independence of the primary nurses on her ward.

One solution might be to abolish the ward sister/charge nurse role and replace it with an administrative officer responsible for supplies, support services, staffing levels and other such areas. The primary nurses then operate as a team of equals responsible for care. The rest of the staff need managing however – bank/agency registered nurses who only act as associate nurses, auxiliaries and of course any students who may be on the ward, be they rostered or supernumerary. The ward administrator could manage these staff in terms of off-duty, annual leave etc., leaving the primary nurses free to be primary nurses.

There is no reason why this development should stop there however. If primary nurses are not managerially responsible to the ward administrator, who are they responsible to, apart from the UKCC and the patient? The intriguing question arises as to whether NHS trusts in the future would want nursing staff as direct employees or even if nurses want to be tied to such a contractual obligation. What is there to stop a group of nurses forming their own primary nursing collective and tendering for contracts to provide a primary nursing service in a unit? The trust manages the bricks and mortar, the administrative officer everything else except the nursing, but the primary nursing collective is responsible for the care delivered within a primary nursing system. Nurses could set up their own agencies to offer such services, free from NHS constraints, subject only to the conditions of a negotiated contract and agreed quality assurance measures.

This might seem all very fanciful and very much the stuff of dreams or nightmares, depending upon your point of view. However, if primary nursing is pushed to its logical limits in terms of autonomy and the current market-oriented culture of the NHS, such a development is logical. This scenario unfolds because pure primary nursing removes the clinical accountability of the ward sister and hence her *raison d'être* in the present system.

If the scenario sketched above is to be avoided, the ward sister's role has to be defined anew. Nursing could follow the medical model and make the sister the primary nurse for all patients on the ward (the named nurse, as s/he currently is in most cases) and thus occupying a similar position to the medical consultant. Staff nurses could then occupy positions akin to registrars and senior registrars, given a large degree of autonomy, but not total autonomy. They are still accountable to the boss. This is an adaptation of primary nursing which might offend the purists as staff nurses become 'semiprimary' nurses or 'secondary' nurses; however, it resolves the dilemma of clinical responsibility. The ward sister could then develop a consultancy role similar to that seen in medical practice with a strong teaching and research component.

The roles of clinical supervisor, professional adviser or consultant, facilitator and teacher are increasingly being explored by ward sisters in primary nursing environments today. These optimistic signs suggest that primary nursing is capable of enhancing the ward sister's role and should not therefore be feared.

Such a change could really see nursing growing a generation of clinical leaders able to exercise power and authority in nursing care, breaking the cycle of learned helplessness discussed earlier. It is easy to see such nurses engaging in meaningful reflection upon practice with staff nurses and developing nursing knowledge out of practice. The writings of authors such as Schon (1983) and Benner (1984) have been extensively referred to elsewhere and really come alive in this approach. The development of such knowledge and its transfer to others within an empowering climate also comprise the key to liberation that has been passionately argued for by Freire (1985). Nursing can achieve liberation by such a route. Primary nursing can empower nurses and demolish hierarchies. Nurses must beware, however, re-creating the same hierarchies on a small scale and destroying nursing leadership by inadvertently making the pivotal ward sister role redundant in their pursuit of primary nursing.

Primary nursing and patient empowerment

Empowerment as a concept should apply equally to patients and nurses if nursing is to liberate itself. There is a large amount of encouraging evidence that primary nursing is associated with patient empowerment, a key component of Mead's description of primary nursing. However the issue remains that staff commitment to a patient-centred approach has to exist before primary nursing can be implemented in its fullest sense.

A good example is provided by the work of Bond *et al.* (1991) who compared a primary nursing ward with a ward which nominally practised team nursing. The primary nursing ward was reported to show much greater patient choice, as shown by details such as a wider range of times for eating meals, getting up and going to bed. There was a wider range of washing and bathing facilities and patients chose when they wanted to use the toilet. Patients were much more involved in care-planning, discussion on medication and decision-taking about future activities. The primary nursing ward showed far less evidence of ward routines and the repetitive meaningless comments which are such a blight upon care plans, while much more effort was made to accommodate the patient's normal home routines.

McMahon's study was also able to demonstrate significant differences in patient involvement. He noted that on a traditionally organized and a team nursing ward, nurses at handover rarely identified and discussed patient problems. When they did identify a problem the usual reaction was either to refer it to someone else, such as a therapist, or ignore it. On the two primary nursing wards observed, one ward featured a detailed handover between staff in the presence of the patient who regularly contributed to the discussion: patient involvement with the opportunity for empowerment was therefore apparent. The other designated primary nursing ward showed a handover pattern similar to the two more traditional wards with no real attempt at patient involvement or

problem-solving. Because a ward has a primary nursing organizational mode does not necessarily mean that the philosophy of
primary nursing is being implemented therefore.

Involvement of the patient in care-planning is facilitated if the
primary nurse ensures the care plan is actually lodged with the
patient. Ahmed and Alarcon (1992) have described such a system in
use with primary nursing and feel it helps discourage the passivity
associated with the sick role and therefore promotes real and active
patient involvement in care-planning.

These studies show evidence of patient empowerment associated
with primary nursing. The study by McCormack (1992) did
however reveal a potential problem in the closeness of the
nurse–patient relationship. It should first be remembered that
McCormack's study involved an in-depth investigation, using
ethnographic techniques, of the views of only four primary nurses
on one ward. It would therefore be unwise to generalize too much
from such a limited sample and replication of his study elsewhere
would be invaluable. Despite that caveat, the interesting finding of
McCormack was the intense sense of ownership by the nurses of
their patients and a reluctance to let go of them. This also extended
to staff acting as associate nurses. The result was that staff only
offered to help other staff when specifically asked to; there was a
lack of the normal spontaneity that characterizes ward work.
McCarthy (1991) also reported major difficulties in implementing
primary nursing in an emergency department in the USA
stemming from this problem of ownership, leading to a break-
down in normal teamwork. A similar problem was identified by
Sella (1991) in reporting on a change to primary nursing in two
medical and two surgical wards.

If staff become possessive about 'their' patients, this can have
other unhealthy effects besides adversely influencing their relationships with other nurses. The nurse as advocate role is undermined
because if the relationship becomes too close, how can the nurse
objectively act as the patient's advocate? Alternatively, who
intercedes on the patient's behalf if the problem requiring advocacy
is the primary nurse?

Empowerment of the patient involves recognizing the patient as
an independent human being, not something that is owned by the
nurse. Phrases such as *My Patient, My Nurse* (Wright 1990) are very
unhelpful as they tend to encourage this kind of dependence and
ownership. The patient is a person, not 'my' anything. This sense of

ownership will therefore undermine one of the basic tenets of primary nursing and what we have called liberation nursing – empowerment of the patient.

It might be that the lack of attention paid to the social sciences in traditional nurse training is partly to blame. It has produced generations of nurses without the benefits of insight into the way people think and behave, particularly when under the stressful conditions imposed by ill health. A great deal of work has to go into communication and counselling skills if nurses are to cope with these stresses and strains as in the past the ritualization of nursing care and its fragmentation into tasks have provided a major defence against such stress for nurses (Walsh and Ford, 1989). Primary nursing involves staff getting much closer to patients and therefore nursing education must equip nurses with the tools to handle new types of patient–nurse relationships. Counselling and communication skills are not learned overnight. The danger is that unprepared nurses may go from one extreme to the other, from fragmentation and distancing the patient to enveloping and internalizing all the individual's problems. A nurse should neither have Teflon skin nor become an enormous sponge, soaking up all 'his' or 'her' patients' problems. This will create an intolerable burden for the nurse to carry.

Primary nursing offers an opportunity to equalize the relationship between nurse and patient. It can redress the balance of power, allowing patients to have the confidence to assert their rights and make known their choices.

If primary nursing empowers the patient that is highly desirable; however, nursing education must equip the nurse to cope with the much closer relationships that will be involved. Nurses must be on their guard against feeling that they own patients – there is no such thing as 'my' patient. Slavery was abolished 200 years ago; nobody owns anybody.

This chapter so far has dwelt at length upon the relationship between empowerment and hierarchy and primary nursing. It is necessary to move on therefore to some of the other characteristics of liberation nursing that were summarized on p. 90, starting with the importance of reflecting upon practice. The continuity of care that primary nursing involves greatly facilitates such activity as the nurse can follow a patient's progress from day to day. The care plan could come to resemble a reflective diary, providing the nurse records his or her own feelings, particularly about critical incidents.

Benner's (1984) arguments for the growth of nursing knowledge out of nursing practice carry a great deal of conviction if nurses are planning and documenting care on a continual basis. The quality of care plans therefore becomes a major issue and also cause for concern as they currently leave a great deal to be desired in many cases. Girvin (1991) has written of the difficulties encountered in implementing primary nursing if care plans are of a poor quality – a view supported by writers such as Bowers (1989). In the absence of the primary nurse, there is only the care plan to work from and if this is a sketchy, out-of-date document couched only in vague generalities, then care will suffer and reflection upon care using such a document will become a meaningless exercise.

A description of care given is not however reflection upon practice. There has to be analysis and questioning and discussion with other colleagues about patient progress which should be open yet unthreatening. The experience gained from nursing patients needs to be shared amongst the ward team – another reason for getting away from the narrow and restrictive 'my patient, my nurse' approach. The nurse must not feel frightened that colleagues will criticize care in a destructive way. Pointing a finger and saying 'You should have done this, not that' is not the way to proceed. Group sessions such as this could be invaluable but would need careful facilitating in order that they achieve their full empowering potential. Perhaps this is a role for the redefined primary nursing ward sister, referred to earlier. Ahmed and Alarcon (1992) have commented on how primary nursing has helped the ward team question their own level of awareness of care and to do so in an atmosphere of openness and trust, the very ideal of empowered and liberated nursing.

Reflection upon practice within a primary nursing environment not only has the potential to meet Benner's requirement that theory should develop out of practice, but also demonstrates the value of the clinical nurse. This latter point is crucial for, as we have noted, much of nursing excellence remains invisible as a result of its preventive nature. Critique of and reflection upon care allow the clinical nurse to demonstrate the effects of nursing intervention in a visible way not possible before. The new-style ward sister becomes the clinical leader and ward manager. S/he can engage in action research with the staff nurses, generating new ideas which can be tested in the real world of clinical nursing from which they came rather than the abstractions of theory where, for example, nursing models are still largely located. There is a burning need to test such models out in practice. Primary nursing might yet provide such a testing ground.

The use of research findings, rather than doing things because that is the way we have always done them, is essential if the nurse is held accountable for practice. If the nurse is indeed called to account for his or her practice and can only offer outmoded care that may be positively contraindicated by research, then in the future employers may consider that as grounds for dismissal. Quality assurance methods may monitor outcomes by named primary nurse and if, for example, patients who had nurse x as their primary nurse are shown to develop twice as many pressure sores as other patients, nurse x will be called to account. Primary nursing allows management to be very specific in monitoring the quality of care. This is something that will be new to nurses for, up to now when things have gone wrong, blame can be dissipated amongst the whole nursing team. In a primary nursing system, the individual nurse will have to stand up and be counted and a lack of a sound rationale for care delivered will be a very serious affair.

The bias for flexibility and action along with changing by doing (praxis) are implicit within primary nursing but not spelt out in Mead's list. The involvement of the patient in care-planning, for example, demands flexibility whilst the involvement of the primary nurse in giving care implies action. The nagging doubt remains though that the organizational mode of primary nursing could be set up but the care that followed would remain unaltered if the deeper philosophical aspects of care are not tackled. A major weakness of all the research mentioned so far which has looked at primary nursing which appears to be working successfully is that it makes no mention of the ward *before* primary nursing was implemented. We return to the theme that primary nursing is really a codification of good nursing practice and therefore flexibility, action, changing by doing will not occur on a ward implementing primary nursing, if certain other predisposing factors are missing.

To implement primary nursing, Girvin (1991) has stressed the need for a lengthy period prior to making any change in which to unfreeze old attitudes. Sella's (1991) study also began with an unfreezing stage as staff explored problems of high turnover and low morale on their wards. She felt this facilitated the change to primary nursing in her study. Girvin is right in talking about proceeding cautiously and of the need for an unfreezing process;

however, she is wrong to talk of unfreezing attitudes before change. The earlier discussion (p. 64) demonstrated that unfreezing consists of establishing the need for change, showing the weaknesses of the present system and involving everybody in this process. Attitudes are more likely to be altered by the experience of implementing the change to primary nursing (cognitive dissonance theory).

The importance of changing attitudes is underlined by Vaughan in an interview with Cole and Davidson (1992), in which she points out that structural change without attitude change will be disastrous, as will rushing into change. Simply putting the visible primary nursing structures in place is not enough. A whole system of working has to be unfrozen and shown to be in need of change. All the staff have to be involved in moving to the new philosophy of care; there is no room for opt-outs. Ahmed and Alarcon (1992) cite their own initial failure at introducing primary nursing as being due to only a partial approach. In the process of change, long-held attitudes and beliefs must be challenged and scrutinized in the light of the experience of working with the new system. Only in this way will the implementation of primary nursing be possible. In other words, there has to be a climate that is receptive to change and that is consistent with the ideas encapsulated within primary nursing.

The key piece of research that is missing, however, is whether primary nursing can transform a poor ward into a good ward. Armitage *et al.* (1991) started off with such a study in mind, investigating the impact of primary nursing on two long-stay psychiatric wards. However, their research involved major structural changes and considerable improvements to the ward conditions, education and training packages for the staff and a deliberate enhancement of the prestige of the wards in question. In light of these intervening variables, it is impossible to say if any improvements that occurred were because of the primary nursing approach or any of the other factors. As we shall see shortly, this is a common criticism which can be levelled at much research which claims to show the merits of primary nursing.

Does primary nursing make any difference?

The nursing literature is overwhelmingly in favour of primary nursing and, as the preceding section has shown, it is consistent with many of the principles outlined in the first section of this book. One such principle is that nurses should be able to give rationales for their actions and this includes switching to primary nursing. To say that primary nursing should be implemented because it sounds like a good idea is not good enough. There must be evidence to support such a change. Bowers (1989), for example, is critical of much of the superficial and descriptive literature which surrounds the subject, 'eulogizing its advantages', in his words. He rightly urges the need for some 'penetration of this fog of wishful thinking': this will be our intent in the following pages.

Researchers have tried to gather such evidence most commonly by attempting to measure the effects of primary nursing on staff satisfaction, patient satisfaction or standards of care. Typically, wards which have implemented primary nursing have been compared with wards that have not, using measures of the three variables described above. The results have been very disappointing for the advocates of primary nursing as they have been unable to show any significant improvements which can be unambiguously attributed to primary nursing.

A fundamental problem that has already been highlighted is that of defining primary nursing. The lack of an operational definition of the key independent variable, in this case primary nursing, undermines the validity and reliability of any research. When researchers experiment with a new chemical which they wish to develop into a drug for example – let us call it Agent X – then teams in different laboratories usually use the same drug and mean the same thing when they talk about Agent X. Unfortunately the same cannot be said about primary nursing. Some researchers might be talking about a simple method of organizing care, others a managerial style which makes it easier to decide which nurse is responsible for what and yet others about a whole-care philosophy.

If the definition has become so all-encompassing as some writers believe then what we are really talking about is good nursing care. Consequently a finding that primary nursing has led to an improvement in nursing translates into a statement that good nursing care leads to good nursing care. In stating the obvious we have demonstrated nothing except an ability to state the obvious. Obvious?

A look back into recent history reveals a major review of the early evaluative research undertaken by Giovanetti (1986) who described the results as inconclusive and showing no benefits to care. She criticized much of the work for flawed methodology. A major problem she felt was the confusion that arose between the terms 'satisfaction levels' and 'perceptions' which were frequently inter-changed. She noted authors often explained their inability to demonstrate improvements in terms of primary nursing not having been fully implemented on the wards under investigation. This is either a feeble excuse for not finding the expected outcome or it shows poor research design.

It is worth pausing to ask just what is meant by satisfaction levels anyway. Is such a measure reliable and valid? What does it mean? Satisfaction is like pain: it is what the person says it is and can be influenced by a whole range of factors. How do individuals give a meaningful overall rating of job satisfaction if some aspects of their job are very satisfying but others quite the opposite?

The very general, subjective nature of the term satisfaction makes it very prone to halo effects. A score of 4 out of 5 for job satisfaction is made up of many components besides the narrow aspect of satisfaction with the job. A nurse may score 4 out of 5 on a satisfaction rating today because she feels good about finishing decorating the dining room and 1 out of 5 tomorrow because of a leak in the plumbing that has just brought the dining-room ceiling down. Either way, her job satisfaction rating has little to do with work or primary nursing.

By virtue of its ability to change rapidly, satisfaction is a potentially unstable measure and therefore lacking reliability, whilst the probability that any rating can reflect all sorts of other factors besides job satisfaction undermines its validity, i.e. the extent to which it is measuring what it says it is. A further problem according to Giovanetti (1986) concerns the difficulty of trying to capture this nebulous concept of job satisfaction in a reliable and valid measuring tool.

Research into staff opinions about primary nursing suffers from a further handicap if the researcher is well-known to the staff as this may influence the results of interviews. For example, MacGuire and Botting (1990) have reported a very favourable opinion of primary nursing amongst a small sample of 10 trained staff on a primary nursing ward when interviewed about the system. However, the researcher carrying out the interviews had worked as a sister and research and development officer in the unit and was known as a keen advocate of primary nursing. It is difficult to see how this did not influence the results.

In this study, the ward was part of a bigger investigation into primary nursing. The sample of nurses for this paper selected themselves as their implementation of primary nursing had received criticism in a local press report and in the words of the researchers: 'The nursing staff on the ward concerned were upset and wanted the opportunity to put on record what they thought about the change'. This gives the impression that the outcomes of the interviews were known in advance. The sample could not be called representative either. These constitute two fundamental weaknesses. McCormack's (1992) study suffers from similar problems as he investigated the perceptions of staff about primary nursing on his own ward. Staff objected to this at a ward meeting and eventually an independent interviewer was brought in to carry out the staff interviews, although McCormack carried out the observational part of the study and was known to the staff as a keen advocate of primary nursing and as the person who would be analysing their interviews. The data gathered are therefore likely to be influenced directly or indirectly by the researcher.

Where a team leader or ward sister tries to measure such a subjective phenomenon as their own staff's job satisfaction concerning a system of nursing with which the researcher is closely identified, the findings must be treated with great caution and the reliability of the findings is open to question.

Staff satisfaction ratings of primary nursing may also depend upon which staff are asked. Sella's (1991) study of four medical surgical wards illustrates this point as, while 100% of those employed as primary nurses agreed with the statement that primary nursing had improved the quality of care, only 53% of associate nurses agreed. Relying upon such a subjective measure as staff opinions which were ascertained with a questionnaire that had not been piloted and which also achieved only a 54% return rate as evidence in favour of primary nursing is very unwise. These sort of methodological difficulties plague and invalidate many claims that research supports the introduction of primary nursing, as we shall see later.

Another problem with evaluating primary nursing by satisfaction measures arises when patient satisfaction is considered. To what extent will the patient give true answers to the questions asked and to what extent will the patient give the answer that s/he thinks is expected to keep everybody happy? There is a real danger that whatever system is being researched, patients will express satisfaction with care partly out of fear of being labelled ungrateful and partly out of a lack of knowledge of anything better.

MacDonald (1988) has raised these issues in her review of the literature on patient satisfaction, pointing out that studies commonly 'suffer' from very high ratings whatever system is being evaluated. In addition to the points advanced above to explain this problem, MacDonald suggests that once again the concept of satisfaction is so nebulous that it is very difficult to define in any meaningful way and that the instruments which have been used simply have not been sensitive enough.

There is a fundamental assumption in measuring patient satisfaction as an index of the success of primary nursing, which is that satisfaction is linked to the system used for the delivery of care. It may not be as Haile (1991) has pointed out, citing the finding of Hamera and O'Connell (1981) that over a 5-day period of study the average amount of time spent by qualified nurses with any one patient totalled 2.25 hours. This is less than half-an-hour a day and worked out at an average of only 2 minutes per interaction.

Proponents of primary nursing would argue that the system increases the amount of time spent with patients. However, Gardner (1991) reports this is not so, for in her comparative study of team and primary nursing, the two methods of care delivery produced very similar amounts of direct patient care. The need for further research into the amount of direct staff nurse–patient contact remains, if primary nursing is to show it genuinely does increase this dimension of care.

Other factors over which the nurse has no control may influence how patients feel about their stay in hospital and hence how they might rate 'patient satisfaction' (with what? Care? Treatment? Nursing? Different questions give different answers). Poorly prepared food, bathwater that is too cool, drab ward surroundings and many other variables may contribute to a low 'satisfaction' rating which is nothing to do with nursing. Salvage's (1985) argument needs to be remembered that nurses have insufficient control and power over so many aspects of the patient's stay to be held really accountable.

McCormack (1992) has highlighted these methodological difficulties in studies which have claimed to show that primary nursing leads to increased patient satisfaction, while the study of Ventura *et al.* (1982) was unable to show any difference in satisfaction, pointing out the personal nature of the concept of satisfaction and the difficulty of definition. Critical evaluation of the literature suggests there is a lack of positive evidence to demonstrate that primary nursing improves patient satisfaction with care delivered.

If the difficulty of using patient/staff satisfaction as an outcome measure is set aside there remains another major criticism of much research which claims primary nursing to be associated with favourable outcomes. It is not possible to say that the outcomes are due to the primary nursing system. There are many other competing explanations which could explain any observed difference: physical improvements to the surroundings, staff training packages, the ward climate and staff philosophy before primary nursing was introduced may have been very positive anyway, staffing levels, staff attitudes, the nature of the patients being cared for and length of time since change to primary nursing are just a few of many factors which could explain changes in staff/patient satisfaction levels or in any more objective quality measure.

One other very important factor is the well-known Hawthorne effect – simply being involved in a research project affects how people behave. Staff may therefore become more aware of and therefore change their practice as a result of being involved in a research project evaluating primary nursing. Such changes might have nothing whatsoever to do with the primary nursing system.

In attempting to avoid the problems of using satisfaction as a measure and instead use a more objective approach, MacGuire (1991) used the Senior Monitor method of measuring quality of care. She investigated three elderly care wards, one of which switched to primary nursing during the study period. Measures with Senior Monitor were carried out on three occasions which showed that indeed the primary nursing ward significantly improved its score after switching to the new system, indicating a higher quality rating. However, the other two wards in the study also improved their scores despite no changes being made in the system of care delivery.

MacGuire suggests that the act of using Senior Monitor to evaluate the quality of care resulted in staff reappraising practice, with the result that improvements took place. The arguments in favour of the nurse as reflective practitioner which we have advanced elsewhere in this book appear to gain support from MacGuire's research, which shows improvements in the quality of care regardless of type of nursing, providing staff stop and think, engaging in a process of critical reappraisal. This is only one study and there are problems with the use of tools such as Monitor and Senior Monitor, which have already been discussed in Chapter 6.

Nevertheless, the implications are that there is no evidence that primary nursing alone improves quality of care.

According to MacGuire, very little research has been carried out which uses objective quality measures to evaluate primary nursing and that which has, has either been methodologically flawed or failed to demonstrate any difference to care.

One recent major American study (Gardner, 1991) has used the Qualpacs system to measure quality in primary and team nursing situations in medical units using patients with cardiac conditions. The results are disappointing. This study did show a statistically significant higher score for the primary nursing compared to the team nursing wards over a 30-month period. Again, though, the team nursing wards also made statistically significant improvements in their scores but not by the same amount as the primary nursing wards, hence the difference. The importance of reflection upon practice, regardless of organizational mode, is demonstrated again. During the period of this study, however, three of the original four units were moved into new buildings and restructured; the impact of this upon the data is not clear but cannot be ignored.

Haile (1991) reminds researchers that if they take this approach they should not include in their quality score any measures which refer to specific characteristics of primary nursing, such as nurses being allocated specific patients to care for, as this introduces bias in favour of the primary nursing ward.

The researchers also report (Gardner, 1991) that the primary nursing units had a much higher proportion of graduate nurses and also had better staff retention rates. The question of intervening variables offering competing explanations for the apparent improvement in care arises again. Do the primary nursing wards score higher because they have better staff retention and a more highly qualified workforce, rather than using a primary nursing system? Is it the primary nursing system that attracts more graduates and improves staff retention, so that the effect of primary nursing on quality of care is indirect? The direct cause of improved quality is the staff.

Other aspects of care were investigated but the researchers could find no difference in staff stress ratings, how the patients rated the amount of support received from staff and how stressful the patients found being in hospital. Primary nursing made no difference to these important measures.

Gardner concludes by pointing out the problems of generalizing from one specific care setting to others in terms of interpreting the limited results she found. She admits that research in a natural clinical setting cannot be carefully controlled, which explains the lack of positive findings, and goes on to observe that it is the philosophical premises of primary nursing which are critical and which should be the focus of future research.

These findings are very typical of much of the research and have led authors such as Haile to question the appropriateness of the experimental design in investigating primary nursing. Where it is impossible to have the tight control over variables that may be exerted in the laboratory and where there are so many possible influences on care, and where measuring outcomes is so subjective and imprecise, this experimental methodology is leading up a blind alley. Add to this the lack of clarity about just what is being researched when people talk of primary nursing, and the position becomes very unsatisfactory.

If the arguments of writers such as Haile, Gardner and MacGuire are developed, they point towards research which looks at the philosophy of primary nursing, trying to discover what nurses mean by it and how various components of this philosophy influence care. The approach of researchers such as Benner (1984) who become involved with the clinical setting and developed theory out of practice is more fruitful than trying to carry out experiments that cannot produce meaningful results.

Nurses should be encouraged to reflect critically upon what they mean by concepts such as patient-centred nursing practice and how they translate such concepts into practice. In this way the key tenets of the emerging philosophy of primary nursing can be identified and the superficial trappings of political gimmickry such as 'the named nurse' dispensed with. Adams and Hardey (1992) have called primary nursing a 'panacea' and warned nurses about the consequences of unthinking uncritical acceptance of an operational mode of questionable long-term benefit. We can only agree with these sentiments. It is in the philosophy of patient-centred care that the real potential benefits to nursing lie, rather than the narrowness of the 'my patient, my nurse' approach.

Conclusions

In this chapter we have taken a critical view of primary nursing rather than the often descriptive and relatively superficial account which may be frequently found in the UK literature, particularly since the Prime Minister's electorally convenient named nurse initiative. In asking the question 'What's in a name?', the reader should remember the rest of the couplet from *Romeo and Juliet*: 'that which we call a rose by any other name would smell as sweet'. In other words, you do not have to be a named nurse or a primary nurse to be a good nurse.

Primary nursing is seen by some as a means of organizing care, by others as a managerial means of calling nurses to account for care given and by many, in a much wider sense, as a whole philosophy of care. These different meanings make it essential that the nurse who wishes to adopt primary nursing knows exactly what is meant by the label 'primary nursing'. Otherwise the nurse is buying a pig in a poke.

If the wider, more philosophical understanding of the term is taken rather than narrow organizational interpretations, primary nursing has many of the characteristics which could help liberate nursing. There is no unambiguous research evidence to support the claim that primary nursing *per se* is better for patients or nurses, however. A more sophisticated approach than simple experiments with organizational models is required, especially when they are usually methodologically flawed. Rather it is about investigating in the real world of nursing what nurses are doing and picking out excellence so that a model (or models) can be built of what nurses mean by patient-centred nursing care. Pat Benner pointed the way in her pioneering work in the 1980s.

Unthinking acceptance of an organizational mode will lead to the ritualization of care, whether that model is called primary nursing or any other form of nursing. Patient care has been improved by good nursing leadership (Whelan, 1988) and also by critical self-appraisal as a result of quality assurance work, as we showed in Chapter 6. Nurses in this way improve practice by critical reflection upon practice, the opposite of ritualistic care.

Primary nursing does not guarantee that a ward will see the back of rituals. Changing the organizational mode of the ward does not stop nurses putting salt in the bathwater or adopting an unthinking ritualistic approach to wound dressings. If attempted change to primary nursing is handled badly, little of benefit will occur and old practices will continue. Critical reflection on practice in an empowering ward climate is essential if organizational changes are to be accompanied by real changes in practice.

Primary nursing itself can become a ritual if nurses are not continually appraising what they are doing and asking if they can do things differently. Care plans can stagnate and initiative wither on the vine if stimulating leadership is lacking. The very nature of what is meant by the phrase 'primary nursing' needs to be addressed as nurses explore the philosophy with which they are working and its implications. This is particularly so because of its possibly disastrous effects upon the ward sister role. An empowering approach would greatly benefit nurses in a primary nursing ward and on a wider scale remove the risk of élitism that may surround the subject. As Finch (1991) has observed, primary nursing has been presented as a 'superior' system used by 'superior' nurses on 'superior' units.

There are fundamental issues of power involved which overshadow issues of nursing accountability and autonomy. Resolution in favour of nursing of the tensions set up by the existence of nurses as an oppressed class must precede a real move towards the philosophy of primary nursing. It may be that primary nursing will help facilitate this shift in power which in turn will help further development of primary nursing. Such a feedback loop would be a major breakthrough in liberating nursing from its current sense of oppression and frustration – ripe breeding grounds for charismatic false messiahs who have the answer to everybody's problems with their 'big idea'. Primary nursing, as Adams and Hardey (1992) have said, is no panacea.

References

Adams A, Hardey M (1992) Primary panacea. *Nursing Times* **88**: 26, 34–35.
Ahmed D, Alarcon A (1992) Whose plan is it anyway? *Nursing Times* **88**: 1, 60.
Armitage P, Champney-Smith J, Andrews K (1991) Primary nursing and the role of the preceptor in changing long-term mental health care; an evaluation. *Journal of Advanced Nursing* **16**: 413–422.
Benner P (1984) *From Novice to Expert*. Menlo Park, Addison Wesley.
Beyer J (1981) Interpersonal communication as perceived by nurse educators in collegial relations. *Nursing Research* **30**: 111–117.
Bond S, Fowler P, Fall M (1991) Evaluating primary nursing part 1. *Nursing Standard* **5**: 36, 35–39.

Bond S, Fowler P, Fall M (1991) Evaluating primary nursing part 2. *Nursing Standard* **5**: 37, 37–39.

Bowers L (1989) The significance of primary nursing. *Journal of Advanced Nursing* **14**: 13–19.

Cole A, Davidson L (1992) Let's name names. *Nursing Times* **88**: 11, 24–26.

Finch M (1991) The steady advance of a revolution. *Nursing Times* **87**: 17, 67–68.

Freire P (1985) *The Politics of Education; Culture, Power and Liberation*. New York, Macmillan.

Gardner K (1991) A summary of findings of a 5 year comparison of primary and team nursing. *Nursing Research* **40**: 113–117.

Giovanetti P (1986) Evaluation of primary nursing. In: Weiley H, Fitzpatrick J, Taunton R (eds) *Annual Review of Nursing Research*, Vol. 4. New York, Springer, pp 127–151.

Girvin J (1991) Implementing primary nursing. *Nursing* **4**: 22–23.

Haile C (1991) Evaluating a change to primary nursing: some methodological considerations. *Nursing Practice* **4**: 12–16.

Hamera B, O'Connell K (1981) Patient centred variables in primary and team nursing. *Research in Nursing and Health* **4**: 183–192.

Hewstone M, Antaki C (1988) Attribution theory and social explanations. In: Hewstone M, Sroebe W, Codol JP, Stephenson G (eds) *Introduction to Social Psychology*. Oxford, Blackwell.

McCarthy M (1991) Implementing a new clinical coordinator role to facilitate primary nursing care; one emergency department's experience. *Journal of Emergency Nursing* **17**: 204–211.

McCormack B (1992) A case study identifying nursing staff's perception of the delivery method of nursing care in practice on a particular ward. *Journal of Advanced Nursing* **17**: 187–197.

MacDonald M (1988) Primary nursing, is it worth it? *Journal of Advanced Nursing* **13**: 797–806.

MacGuire J (1991) Quality of care assessed: using the Senior Monitor index in three wards for the elderly before and after a change to primary nursing. *Journal of Advanced Nursing* **16**: 511–520.

MacGuire J, Botting D (1990) The use of the ethnograph program to identify the perceptions of nursing staff following the introduction of primary nursing in an acute medical ward for elderly people. *Journal of Advanced Nursing* **15**: 1120–1127.

McMahon R (1990) Power and collegial relations among nurses on wards adopting primary nursing and hierarchical ward management structures. *Journal of Advanced Nursing* **15**: 232–239.

Manthey M (1980) *The Practice of Primary Nursing*. Oxford, Blackwell.

Mead D (1991) An evaluation tool for primary nursing. *Nursing Standard* **6**: 1, 37–39.

Peterson C, Seligman M (1984) Causal explanations as a risk factor for depression: theory and evidence. *Psychological Review* **91**: 347–374.

Salvage J (1985) *The Politics of Nursing*. Oxford, Butterworth-Heinemann.

Schon D (1983) *The Reflective Practitioner*. New York, Basic Books.

Seligman M (1975) *Helplessness*. San Francisco, Freeman.

Sella S (1991) One year later, evaluating a change in delivery system. *Nursing Forum* **26**: 5–11.

Thomas L (1992) Qualified nurse and nursing auxiliary perceptions of their work environment in primary, team and functional nursing wards. *Journal of Advanced Nursing* **17**: 373–382.

Ventura M, Fox R, Corley M, Mercurino S (1982) A patient satisfaction measure as a criterion to evaluate primary nursing. *Nursing Research* **31**: 226–230.

Walsh, M Ford P (1989) *Nursing Rituals; Research and Rational Action.* Oxford, Butterworth-Heinemann.

Whelan J (1986) Ward sisters' management styles and their effects on nurses' perceptions of quality of care. *Journal of Advanced Nursing* **13**: 125–138.

Wright S (1990) *My Patient, My Nurse.* London, Scutari.

8 *The nurse practitioner*

Before discussing the possible contribution that the nurse practitioner (NP) may make to the liberation of nursing, it is necessary to review the origins of the concept and outline what is meant by the term 'nurse practitioner'. In general terms, an NP is a nurse who operates autonomously: he or she is largely independent of doctors and fully accountable for his or her actions. The extended role of the nurse debate in the UK has for many years hindered the development of the NP. This concept has now fortunately been replaced by the UKCC document *The Scope of Professional Practice*, which paves the way for the removal of many petty local restrictions and their replacement with the general principle of accountability for actions carried out (UKCC, 1992).

In considering the NP role, the guiding principles are the UKCC *Scope of Professional Practice* and *Code of Professional Conduct* documents and the legal principle that the nurse should only work within his/her level of competence and skill unless in a dire emergency, and at all times take reasonable care and precautions (Dimond, 1990). This has clear implications for education and training in the NP role, as a nurse carrying out activities for which s/he has not been prepared is acting outside the UKCC code of conduct and will almost certainly fall foul of either the criminal or civil law eventually. Dimond points out that at all times the nurse is accountable to the UKCC, the law (both civil and criminal) and to his/her employer, in addition of course to him- or herself. In considering the NP role, these rigorous rules of accountability need to be remembered at all times.

The development of nurse practitioners in North America

In the mid 1960s, the USA faced a shortage of doctors providing primary care, particularly in inner-city and remote rural areas. This stimulus, as well as the perennial problems of escalating costs, gave rise to the NP concept, along with the allied development of physician's assistants. The initial focus of NPs was upon assessment and management of patients in primary care, using some techniques of assessment, for example, that were traditionally the preserve of the medical profession. Despite initial resistance from the nursing authorities in the USA on the grounds that this development would lead to nurses taking on medical tasks which were inappropriate and dangerous, this initiative quickly gathered momentum such that in 1974 there were 87 certificate programmes offering training. By 1980 over half of these training programmes were at Masters degree level and by 1981 there were over 14 000 NPs in the USA (Bowling and Stilwell, 1988).

A recent review of the role of the NP by Huch (1992) summarizes most training programmes as focusing on assessment and communication skills, health promotion and disease prevention, the management of chronic illness and also the medical management of patients. This is essential to meet the five main domains of practice identified by Huch:

1.   Management of the client's health/illness status.
2.   Monitoring and ensuring the quality of health-care practice.
3.   Organization of care and role competencies.
4.   The teaching and coaching function of the nurse.
5.   The healing role of the nurse.

This latter area of practice does not preclude the NP from terminal care for, as Benner and Wrubel (1989) point out, allowing patients to make sense of their illness, even if it eventually may prove fatal, is a form of healing as it reverses the loss of self-understanding and alienation that accompany illness.

The exact functions vary from state to state but typically include thorough assessment, including a complete physical examination using techniques which used to be thought of as purely medical, such as chest auscultation; ordering laboratory tests and X-rays; performing minor surgery, including local anaesthetic infiltration; prescribing and dispensing medication from stock and independently assessing and managing client caseloads. The nurse can act on her or his own judgement, only referring to a doctor when necessary.

Huch (1992) considers that there are significant differences from the physician's assistant role as the NP is an autonomous and independent health-care worker. The physician's assistant, despite a degree-level training, still works closely under the physicians's orders within a task-focused structure. By contrast, the NP must have a theory-based conceptual framework to guide practice and can practise independently, but in collaboration with the physician. However, this independence is somewhat of an illusion, as the NP needs medical authorization to perform many of the medically related functions that have become part of her/his role. It is perhaps more accurate to describe the NP as semiautonomous in that, while some of the aspects of the role are truly autonomous, significant others require medical authorization to practise.

The situation is further complicated by the current crisis in health care in the USA which has led many physicians to express opposition to NPs for fear of unemployment. The medical shortages of the 1960s have abated and, although the 1970s were marked by increased acceptance of the NP role, the late 1980s have seen the growing perception that they constitute a threat to the employment prospects of doctors (Bowling and Stilwell, 1988).

Restrictions on their role and interference in practice have led many NPs to set up in independent practice as nurse entrepreneurs (Slauenwhite, 1991), functioning outside the state-run health-care system. Although this brings with it all the problems of managing a business in addition to the NP role, it does free the nurse from the inevitable limitations associated with any large organization, subject of course to whatever limits state legislation imposes.

The picture that emerges in North America is that nursing developed its scope sufficiently to claim true professional autonomy for substantial areas of theory-based practice and a delegated autonomy for other complementary areas. This was underpinned by educational advancement up to higher degree level, with most of the development occurring in primary health care, although as we shall see later, hospital emergency departments (Accident and Emergency; A&E) have also proved fertile ground for the development of this role.

There is little doubt that the value of the NP role has been supported by a very impressive collection of research demonstrating the benefits to patients of the NP consultation. This has been summarized by Ventura (1988), who reviewed the American literature between 1963 and 1983, analysing 248 reports on NPs. They are found most commonly in community-care areas and perform a comprehensive range of activities which greatly expand nursing practice, as well as replacing some of the work previously done by doctors. The review showed that the NPs carried out these activities at least as well as other health-care professionals, including doctors – and sometimes better. They had beneficial effects upon patient outcomes, particularly in areas such as compliance with treatment regimes for chronic health problems, health promotion and maintenance.

A further major study by Ventura (1988) also showed a high degree of job satisfaction amongst NPs related to independence of practice and their interreactions with clients in the delivery of care. Ventura concludes from this extensive review of the North American literature that NPs should be supported as a very effective means of health-care delivery, particularly in the community and in the management of clients with long-term health-care problems. The NP could, for example, play a major role in meeting the increasing health-care needs of the elderly. The success of the NP seems well-established, so much so that future research might be directed not so much to evaluating their impact any further, but to asking why are they so successful?

Nurse practitioners in the UK

In the UK, tracing the development of the NP has been made difficult by the proliferation of titles used to describe the concept. Clinical nurse specialist (CNS), nurse practitioner, advanced practitioner, practice nurse, specialist nurse, consultant nurse and even supernurse are all terms which occur in the literature. However, the very positive patient outcomes demonstrated in the USA make the NP concept worthy of investigation in the UK.

A major early attempt to explore this area was carried out by Castledine (1982) who focused on the CNS title and tried to discover what common features there were amongst nurses in posts entitled CNS. He found little consensus, as the title appeared to cover a very wide range of responsibilities; however, it was possible to differentiate CNS staff into two broad categories – those who had specialist knowledge related to specific technical skills and those who had a broader, more in-depth knowledge base. In either case, they were more effective when allowed to practise across a range of settings wherever care was needed rather than restricted to one area.

Markham (1988) has written of the need to develop the CNS role by adding research, teaching and management skills to the clinical component in such a way that the CNS becomes a nursing leader and a change agent. In her view a nurse is a CNS only if involved in all of these functions. She acknowledges the difficulty of this, describing how many CNS staff that she could identify were carrying out little original nursing research; instead they were mostly supporting medical research and product trials. This led Markham to appoint a director of nursing research within her hospital (the Royal Marsden) to upgrade this aspect of CNS functioning.

Even if the rounded picture of the CNS presented by Markham is accepted as a blueprint for NP growth, there has been considerable disagreement about the areas into which the NP may develop and other characteristics of their role. Barker (1988) pointed out three possible ways that the NP may be defined, the first of which was by relation to a biomedical frame of reference. Stoma therapists, renal nurses and breast-care nurses are examples. An alternative pattern relates to the nature of the nursing work such as counselling or continence promotion, while finally there is the whole health-promotion field of practice (health visitors, school nurses, etc.). It would be a mistake to limit the field and say that only one of these approaches is correct; they are all equally valid, providing the essential characteristics of the NP are present. The problem is that there is, as yet, little UK agreement about what those characteristics are and how they may be achieved, although Barker does suggest an education at further degree level, consistent with the North American approach.

NPs are seen by some as an élite band of nurses. Shuttleworth (1991) described them as high-flyers, pushing back clinical boundaries and taking on ever-increasing responsibilities. She rightly points out that the structures within nursing must change to allow nurses to develop to their full clinical potential. However, the use of the phrase 'supernurse' by Shuttleworth, borrowed from the Prime Minister, John Major, does her argument a disservice as it sounds very élitist and divisive. If the suggestion made by Barker that NP education should be at higher degree level is followed, this too will severely limit the numbers of NPs who will emerge.

An opposing view of NP development comes from Andrews (1988) who discusses the role of a typical community nurse and suggests that this already encompasses many of the characteristics of NPs found in the USA. Andrews goes on to argue that all community staff have the potential to become NPs and that 'Far from becoming the new role of the exclusive few this could become the aspiration of all'.

The UKCC has held back the development of the nurse practitioner by adherence to the extended role of the nurse principle, finally abandoned in 1992 and replaced with the potentially more empowering document 'Scope of Professional Practice' (UKCC, 1992). The extended-role concept and the unimaginative approach of hierarchical nursing management strangled nursing practice with a mass of bureaucratic red tape and certificates. This change in policy, if implemented creatively and responsibly, can greatly facilitate NP development in the UK. Further very welcome developments from the statutory bodies have been initiatives such as the English Nursing Board (ENB) Higher Award which now offers the nurse the chance to support and develop clinical practice with a first-degree-level education.

Future nurses will all be qualifying with at least a Diploma in Higher Education under the Project 2000 system. It is therefore logical that any major educational initiative that takes the nurse beyond registration should be at the next academic level up from diploma, which is at first degree level (BA or BSc). The ENB Higher Award therefore seems an appropriate route for NP preparation and offers a compromise between the élitist, 'supernurse' higher-degree view and the more egalitarian, 'everybody can be NP' view presented earlier. It is still essential, however, for the growth and advancement of the profession, to offer higher degrees in nursing to permit the development of those nurses who, having achieved graduate status, can see areas of development in practice consistent with postgraduate studies and research.

The discussion so far has identified key areas such as research, leadership and staff development and the initiation of change which need to go alongside the clinical component of the NP role. Areas of practice have been identified and education up to first degree level via a clinically focused route such as the ENB Higher Award is suggested as the ideal future preparation. This much consensus can be established. However, the literature reviewed so far has failed to tackle the issue which is at the crux of the matter – professional autonomy. To what extent can the NP distance her- or himself from medical control and also claim to be practising within a coherent theoretical framework? These are the two distinctive components of the NP in North America.

Can the nurse practitioner liberate nursing practice?

It is worth reflecting on the general discussion so far to see what effect the development of the NP movement in the UK might have on the future development of nursing, along the lines outlined in the first section of this book.

On p. 90 we outlined some of the factors which we believe are characteristic of liberation nursing, starting with valuing the nurse and patient. An essential step in establishing the value of the nurse will have been taken if the NP can show s/he has something unique to contribute to the role which another professional cannot. Simply being a doctor's assistant or cheap substitute for the doctor is not enough. There must also be evidence that the patient values the NP whilst the NP sees the patient as a valued individual in his or her own right, rather than another case requiring some technical procedure which used to be done by the doctor. The evidence from North America cited by Ventura is replete with examples of patient satisfaction with the NP service, whilst the guidelines for NP education stress areas such as holistic care and communication skills besides technical aspects of care. This contributes to the valuing of the patient by the practitioner.

The removal of hierarchies from the care system is an essential precursor to the development of the NP role. Managers have to trust the NP and cannot interfere in day-to-day practice. Such interference was cited in Ventura's work (1988) as one of the main causes of concern to NPs. Hierarchical problems also extend across professions and, whilst the obvious group with whom there might be problems are doctors, there are others such as radiographers and other professions allied to medicine. A great deal of work is necessary with the medical profession to overcome a century or more of traditional beliefs about the roles of nurses – and also women – if doctors are to stop treating nurses as inferiors.

Even within the USA it is acknowledged that doctors still exert some control over areas of the NP role. Empowerment is about sharing, therefore nurses who seek empowerment should be able to collaborate with other staff, including doctors. Consequently medical influence on aspects of the NP role may be argued as consistent with empowerment, providing it is upon a more equal footing. Total independence from the medical profession is therefore not necessary, besides probably being unrealistic for the development of the NP role as an empowering and liberating concept.

The NP is in an excellent position to develop the skills of reflective practice. Being responsible for her/his own caseload and working patterns gives the NP the opportunity to follow a range of patients over long periods of time. Thinking about practice while working independently, rather than following orders or carrying out a list of repetitive tasks, fosters the reflective mode of working. If NPs are to be truly accountable for their practice they would ignore research findings at their peril and, as we have seen, there is strong support for the research role of the NP. It should be stressed that this need not be in the formal, empirical style discussed on p. 50 but could involve the use of action research techniques which would be complementary to reflective practice. The NP who brings together these elements of reflective practice, research awareness and action research would, as Benner has argued (1984) develop nursing knowledge in action. In this way nursing can develop its theoretical framework from practice, and such a framework is an essential requirement in the definition of the NP in North America.

NPs working in community care are in an ideal position to work with patients in promoting health. Empowerment of the patient thus becomes a major possible strategy for the NP. It is important to keep notions of élitism at bay within nursing itself, for if NPs were seen as some high-flying supernurses this would be divisive and counter-productive in terms of empowering nurses. Hierarchies are the antithesis of empowerment and, having struggled to be free from the domination of other groups such as managers and doctors, nurses would be defeating the whole object of the exercise if they set up an élite corps within nursing who dominated the rest of the profession. The NP of the future must be seen as a member of the nursing team who, while having a unique contribution to make to patient care, is still a team player. Structures must be such that there is collaboration and mutual respect amongst the nursing team with a sharing of ideas and contributions towards care. In many cases the NP may have more of an outside consultant role rather than a team leader. Either way, regression into the old hierarchical way of working should be carefully avoided.

The importance of education in developing the NP cannot be underestimated. First degree level is suggested as a compromise between an exclusive further degree level and a level which is insufficient to be compatible with the intellectual and academic skills such as analysis, synthesis and practice development in light of reflection which are required by the NP. Education must equip the

NP with more than new technical skills, however important they may be. It must also teach the NP to be inquisitive, reflective and constructively critical in addition to developing communication and interpersonal skills, research, innovative management and leadership skills. If education becomes fixed purely on a medical model the NP initiative will have failed (see Freire's critique (1985) of education as a form of domination, p. 57), as it would if the level was insufficient to equip the nurse to function as an NP.

The educational initiative for NPs has been taken by the Royal College of Nursing (RCN) Institute of Advanced Nursing Education which has started the first NP course in the UK, currently at diploma level. To date the statutory bodies in the UK have been distinctly lukewarm in supporting this initiative and the long-awaited UKCC report on *Post-Registration Education and Practice* dismissed the term 'nurse practitioner' as 'ambiguous and misleading' (Casey, 1993). This report has continued the divisions within community health care by proposing six different areas of community practice. It ignored the chance to unite community health care in the way that the NHS Management Executive (NHSME) outlined in its report *New World, New Opportunities* (1993), published at exactly the same time. The views expressed in the NHSME document were completely at odds with the UKCC and yet both were published in the same week. As Casey (1993) points out, this is clearly absurd and confusing. Is it not beyond the bounds of possibility that the UKCC and the NHSME might actually communicate with each other to try and achieve some degree of consensus before releasing such important documents?

The style of working that is usually associated with an NP offers great scope for flexibility and creativity, providing the educational base is sound and the practitioner is not strangled with management regulations and imposed constraints for which no reasonable rationales are given. The NP role personifies clinical excellence and, with it, the change of practice by doing – nursing praxis.

It can be seen therefore that the NP concept has great potential to fulfil the criteria set out on p. 90 for liberation nursing. On a cautionary note, however, the potential also exists for the NP idea to be devalued. If the NP is not properly educated and prepared, practice could very easily become as fossilized and unresponsive to research as may still be seen in some areas today, particularly if another professional group controls that educational process and uses it for its own benefit so that NPs only learn what the dominant group wishes them to learn. Severe and seemingly arbitrary constraints imposed on practice by management and other professional groups will also lead towards ritualization of care.

Inconsistencies of role function will tend to devalue the NP concept. The situation where a nurse carries out an activity only if the doctor is unavailable, but otherwise the doctor would do it, is not consistent with the role of the NP and trivializes nursing. We have already seen that a great number of titles have been used in the UK literature on NPs and the danger exists of confusion arising as staff use terms with different meanings from other staff. Standardization of nomenclature and clear definitions of the NP are therefore desirable.

It would be a retrograde step for nursing if NPs became an élitist group whose word was accepted unchallenged by other nurses. The hierarchical traditions which we have identified as contributing towards ritualistic nursing would only be propagated in this way. The last thing nursing needs is 'experts' telling other nurses what to do in an authoritative style that precludes challenge and question. Rather NPs should share their expertise as members of a team, recognizing the validity of other staff's points of view, and facilitating the overall development of knowledge within the nursing team. It does not require a great deal of imagination to see how easy it is for an ill-guided NP to become a false messiah!

The impact of the nurse practitioner on care: some examples

The rest of this chapter will look at evaluative studies of experimental schemes involving NPs in both community and accident and emergency settings. The pioneering work in the UK is widely recognized to have been that of Stilwell. She began with some basic questions, such as: could an NP working in a general practitioner (GP) surgery differentiate between medically trivial and more serious conditions and, more importantly, could s/he provide opportunities for health promotion and disease prevention (Stilwell *et al.*, 1988)?

The outcome of this work was a major research project in an inner urban area of North Birmingham which involved Stilwell working as an NP in a surgery where two male GPs worked without the benefit of a practice nurse (Stilwell *et al.*, 1987). The role of the NP coincided with that proposed in the Cumberledge Report (DHSS, 1986) into community nursing services and centred on screening,

health education and advice; maintenance of patient care programmes for the chronically sick; the diagnosis and treatment of
specific diseases within agreed medical protocols; referral on to a
doctor of patients who fell outside the protocols and also referral on
to the community nursing services where appropriate.

A notice in the waiting room described the functions of the NP
and patients were asked by the receptionist whether they wished to
see the doctor or NP. During the period of the study, 858 patients
were seen by the NP. This group spanned the full age range but
there was a marked female bias, women accounting for 72% of the
patients seen. The principal ethnic groups in the NP sample were
UK 73% and New Commonwealth/Pakistan 20%, compared to 92.5
and 2.1% respectively in the local population.

The types of problems presented spanned the whole range of
diagnostic groups but the largest single group, which accounted for
60% of consultations, could best be described as preventive and
health education or advice-giving. Stilwell felt she had acted as an
alternative consultant for patients and notes that 45% of the patients
were managed without prescription, further investigation or
referral. It was possible to develop the health education and
advice-giving part of her role as a result of having 20-minute
consultations rather than the much shorter times that are
characteristic of GPs. It is not accidental that in 46% of consultations
patients introduced extra health problems beyond the first stated
problem that had brought them to the surgery.

This pioneering work clearly demonstrated the feasibility of the
concept of the NP working in the community. However, there were
significant problems with this early piece of work, which were
pointed out by Salisbury and Tettersell (1988), the first of which is
that the environment was not typical. Single-handed GPs are
becoming less frequent as health centres with teams of health-care
staff, including GPs working in group practices, become more the
norm. A second weakness with this work was that it did not
compare the NP's caseload with the doctors'; consequently little
could be concluded regarding any different service utilization by
patients. It was not really possible to answer the question of whether
the NP provided a substitute for the GP or an intrinsically different
service. The facts that 72% of her caseload were women and 20%
were ethnically Pakistani or New Commonwealth are startling, but
in themselves of little significance unless similar figures are available
for GP consultations at the same period.

The final problem with this work concerns the lack of a direct evaluation exercise to explore a patients' feelings about the service. Instead a questionnaire was sent to a random sample of 140 patients on the GP list asking them about their attitudes towards NPs. Just under half of these patients (48%) had had a consultation with the NP. It is worth noting that only 6% of the sample were ethnically New Commonwealth/Pakistani, compared to 20% of the NP caseload, which makes this an unrepresentative sample. The patients who had consulted the NP had different perceptions about her role compared to those who had not. In view of the fundamental difference introduced by the factor of whether the person had seen the NP or not, consideration of the results from this study as if it were only one group of patients is problematical. However, the finding that 53 out of 61 patients who had seen the NP (87%) would be happy to see her again is interesting, although the circumstances under which this would apply are not clear from what was posed as a hypothetical question.

What was of value in this exercise was the qualities picked out by the patients as preferable in somebody they would consult professionally about health problems. The most common were treating the person as an individual (44%), followed by being understanding (35%), the ability to answer questions (23%) and listening carefully (20%). Only 11% mentioned the possession of medical qualifications. The authors suggest that the most common reasons for NP consultation were health education or social and emotional problems and speculate that the patient's perceptions of doctors and nurses may influence which they would choose to see, although they concede they have no evidence to support that suggestion.

Salisbury and Tettersell (1988), mindful of the weaknesses in the pioneering work of Stilwell *et al.*, developed their own study of the impact an NP may make in a more typical group practice in Reading. They introduced the NP in the hope of extending the range of services offered to patients rather than as a means of providing a GP substitute, and the NP role was not defined in terms of tasks, but rather in terms of areas of activity such as health promotion. This study compared the work done by the NP with a GP and also evaluated patient satisfaction (but see p. 116) with the services offered.

Patients attending the health centre were offered the choice of seeing the GP or the NP. There was therefore free choice based upon information made available in the health centre. The NP saw patients of a similar age range and gender distribution to the GP used as comparison. The major difference was that the GP tended to see more patients with new problems and complaints that were more specific, while the NP patients tended to have chronic problems and complaints of a more general nature, such as obesity, hypertension and diabetes. The NP managed 78% of her consultations without referral to a doctor and 89% without resorting to prescribed drugs. Her most common activities were giving advice about weight and diet, management of patients with hypertension, diagnosis of rashes and management of patients with asthma and diabetes. A follow-up questionnaire on 100 patients produced a good response rate (73%), of whom 97% said they would consult the NP again if the need arose.

The authors concluded from this study that the NP provided an intrinsically different service for patients from that offered by the GP and therefore represented an extension of patient choice rather than a GP substitute. Patients formed different relationships with the NP as she offered different attitudes and skills, not having trained with the traditional biomedical model of the doctors. This is consistent with the aim of empowering the patient through choice. Their second conclusion was that patients found it easier to talk to the NP than to the doctor. This might be a simple personality effect or it could be due to longer consultation times or the patient's perception of the nurse. The longer consultation times may well have made for more beneficial consultations, but as the authors point out in their final conclusion, this also means that the NP is not a cheaper alternative to the GP as she sees far fewer patients in a session. They conclude by urging doctors to see the NP as a valuable asset in general practice rather than as a threat to their role.

This study by Salisbury and Tettersell is consistent with the findings of Stilwell *et al.* but offers a more secure base to work from as it was carried out in a more typical primary health-care environment, compares the workload of the NP with a doctor and has good evidence of patient satisfaction. Consideration of this work suggests that the NP role in primary health care is capable of achieving the goal of liberating nursing practice.

It is salutary to note, however, that it is over a decade since Stilwell's pioneering work and little progress has been made in developing the NP role within primary health care, apart from the initiative of Salisbury and Tettersell. It is sad, for example, to read of the immense difficulties experienced by Burke-Masters (1988) in trying to offer an NP service to the homeless in London.

The impact of the government's NHS changes and the introduction of the internal market and fund-holding GPs have overshadowed the development of the NP role in primary health care. To this must be added the Care in the Community changes which are shifting resources away from health care towards social services departments. The traditional suspicion of changes in nursing and medical roles which might have been expected from an inherently conservative medical profession may well have been greatly exacerbated by the wholesale changes in the NHS which the government has enforced upon reluctant doctors and nurses alike.

The long-drawn-out review of community nursing education being undertaken by the UKCC has led to great uncertainty over the whole of the future roles of staff, such as health visitors and district nurses. Community staff have also been absorbed by the skill mix and reprofiling exercises of 1992–1993 which they see as downgrading community nursing. Unfortunately, in all this controversy, the NP concept seems to have got rather lost in arguments about clinical grading and professional rivalries involving health visitors, district and practice nurses.

The NP role offers a way forwards which is in the patient's interest and sadly, amongst all the professional rhetoric, the patient has rather been forgotten. Nurses in the community have many examples of professional excellence set for them by NPs in North America and, as we have seen, in the UK. It is time for change, for moving away from traditionally held professional positions which can no longer be defended until the last ditch. Health visitors, district nurses and practice nurses cannot criticize doctors for holding up change when they themselves cannot come together in the interests of everyone and recognize the need for change. The development of the NP role in the community offers a constructive and professionally enhancing way forwards.

As this book was going to press, the UKCC released its disappointing *Community Education and Practice Proposals* which have met widespread opposition within the profession. This document seems set to propagate the divisions within community health care by opting for no less than six areas of practice, each given the sort of clumsy and bureaucratic title that is the UKCC's trademark. Added to this will be three levels of practice, primary, specialist and advanced, which when combined with the ENB's

Higher Awards should ensure that the average clinical nurse is thoroughly confused. At a time when nursing desperately needs clear and unifying leadership we find that the statutory bodies are at odds with government and each other, and as a result giving nursing just the opposite of what it needs.

The nurse practitioner in hospital

It could be argued that many clinical nurse specialists (e.g. stoma or breast-care nurses) are in large part NPs. There is no doubting the specialist knowledge, technical skills and experience of such nurses. The key questions to be asked, however, in deciding whether a clinical nurse specialist can be called an NP are to what extent is practice independent of medical control? What educational preparation has the person had? To what extent is the person's work following a holistic, health-oriented nursing approach, and is there a theoretical framework within which the person is operating?

The UKCC *Post-Registration Education and Practice report* (1993) puts forward the notion of specialist and advanced levels of practice and dismisses the phrase 'nurse practitioner'. The argument should not be about semantics and titles but about roles and responsibilities. The NP is a concept and it is important to keep that in mind in the debates about the UKCC proposals. To what extent can the characteristics of the NP concept in hospital nursing be picked out of the UKCC pronunciations upon the topic? If the characteristics are there, the title is of secondary importance but if the UKCC intentions are to subvert the principles of largely autonomous nursing practice behind the smokescreen of a title such as 'advanced nursing practice', they are doing nursing a grave disservice.

One of the principal hospital areas in North America where the NP role has been developed has been the Emergency Department (ED), or A&E unit in UK parlance. As interest has been shown in this development by nurses in the UK it is worth comparing examples from both sides of the Atlantic.

A very good account of the development of the role of the NP within an emergency-room setting is provided by Covington and Sellers (1992). Their hospital ED was experiencing increasing demand and ever longer waiting times for patients with minor conditions. Incidentally, this is a consequence of effective triage: in ensuring that the most seriously ill and injured are seen first, the less serious patients logically have to wait longer. The effect of lengthy delays was an increase in complaints and more and more patients walking out untreated. This was leading to a loss in revenue which the ED could not afford.

The solution was an experimental NP-staffed fast-track service for minor conditions staffed by two NPs, with a physician working in the main ED, but to whom they could refer their patients if needed. The greater knowledge base was crucial in appointing NPs rather than registered nurses to these two posts. The job description is given in Figure 8.1 and acts as a useful illustration of what is required of an NP in North America. Triage criteria were developed for allocating patients to the NP fast track. The original opening hours were set for the busiest period in the ED, from 1200 hours Friday until 2200 hours Monday, and it took about 5 months for the NPs to become really proficient and to establish good working relationships with the doctors, based on mutual trust and confidence.

The system proved very successful, with the NPs on duty treating 20 patients per day. Walkout rates halved and the hospital decided to recruit four more NPs and run the NP fast track 7 days a week, 12 hours a day. The NPs recruited were all trained in the primary-health-care NP role and so required an intensive 3-month in-service training package to develop their ED-based skills.

The system has been evaluated internally by peer review, auditing a sample of records, monitoring waiting times for X-rays, carrying out 48-hour post-discharge telephone checks on certain categories of patients such as those with head injuries, and having discussions with nursing and medical staff across the whole ED. Support is widespread for the system as it relieves pressure on the main ED by freeing up staff to work on those patients who most need intensive medical and nursing care and it is also increasing the revenue of the department – a very important consideration in the USA. A survey of a sample of 117 patients produced overwhelming endorsement, with 96% stating that the care they received was either excellent or very good and 98% stating that they would recommend the service to others.

This impressive example of the use of the NP in a hospital setting demonstrates the qualities of liberation nursing that have been discussed elsewhere. Demonstrably high-quality practice with a great deal of autonomy based upon a good educational base is benefiting patients, nurses, doctors and hospital alike.

FAMILY NURSE PRACTITIONER
EMERGENCY DEPARTMENT

I. JOB SUMMARY

The Family Nurse Practitioner is a professional registered nurse with advanced education and training in the primary care of adult and pediatric populations. The Family Nurse Practitioner is responsible for providing primary care to Emergency Department patients under the medical supervision of the Emergency Department Attending physician and as directed by clinical protocols. This responsibility involves ongoing collaboration with Emergency physicians.

II. QUALIFICATIONS:

(a) A Master of Science Degree in nursing, encompassing twelve to twenty-four months of specialized classroom and experiential learning as a nurse practitioner.

(b) One year of related clinical nursing experience.

(c) Professional knowledge of nursing theory and practice. Extensive knowledge of physical assessment, differential diagnosis, pathophysiology, pharmacology and management of acute and chronic patient/family problems.

(d) Current licensure required by the State of Tennessee to practice as a Nurse Practitioner. Certification preferred.

(e) Substantial interpersonal skills necessary to instruct patients and their families and to collaborate with health team members.

III. ACCOUNTABILITY

1. Emergency Department Attending physicians
2. Senior Nurse Practitioner
3. Nursing Director, Emergency Department

IV. RESPONSIBILITIES

A. Clinical

1. Obtains patient histories on Emergency Department patients.
2. Performs physical assessments pertinent to patients' chief complain.
3. Evaluates assessment data and establishes diagnoses.
4. Differentiates patient care situations which require immediate and nonimmediate actions and responds accordingly.
5. Orders and evaluates appropriate diagnostic studies.
6. Performs and monitors therapeutic procedures.
7. Assesses and/or manages follow-up plans.
8. Records and documents assessment data, interventions, results, and patient outcomes.
9. Educates patients and/or their families in order to promote wellness, prevent health problems, maintain current health and intervene in acute or chronic illness.
10. Documents discharge teaching and patient instructions for follow-up.

B. Administrative

1. Facilitates and implements systems which promote and maintain effective communication and collaboration with inter/intra hospital physicians, nurses and other members of the health care team.
2. Maintains appropriate records and documentations of clinical and educational activities.
3. Collaborates with physicians in the development of clinical protocols/procedures for the delivery of in-patient care.
4. Demonstrates ability to work effectively with patients, families and with professional and supportive personnel who provide patient care.
5. Recognizes and uses appropriate channels to communicate stressful patient care/performance situations that arise with physicians, families and other staff members.
6. Collaborates with other nurse practitioners to reach consensual agreement on staffing schedules.

C. Research/Scholarly Activities

1. Identifies the need for and participates in scholarly/research activities.

D. Education

1. Acts as resource to Emergency Department staff and implements educational programs which will improve clinical skills, enhance knowledge base and improve patient care.
2. Maintains and enhances a current level of knowledge relative to professional practice, as well as continuing education requirements necessary for licensure.
3. Accepts self-responsibility for advancing skills and continuing education by:
   a. Setting realistic and measurable goals for individual developmental needs based on personal, peer and supervisory evaluations of strengths and learning needs.
   b. Assessing own performance status in relation to this position description and progress toward achievement of professional goals on an annual basis.
   c. Seeking learning experiences/responsibilities to strengthen areas requiring development and to advance knowledge about other current developments in nursing.

Figure 8.1 *Job description for fast-track nurse practitioners (Covington and Sellers, 1992, reproduced with permission from Mosby-Year Book, Inc.)*

It remains to investigate experiments with the NP role that have been written up in the UK literature. Potter (1990) has described the interest shown by the RCN in this field and gives a definition developed by the RCN A&E Forum (now A&E Association) which stresses autonomy, excellence and nursing-related psychosocial skills besides technical activities. He rightly laments the many good ideas in nursing which have gone sadly wrong as a result of hasty implementation, citing clinical grading and the nursing process as two good examples. Potter is a good advocate for the NP role in A&E, stressing the need for education for practice, but there are two problems with his views.

First, in advocating in-service training as the educational route to NP status he is short-changing the NP and potentially leaving him or her underprepared. A detailed national curriculum for NP education in A&E is not required, but utilization of the ENB Higher Award framework or some parallel development, linked in to higher education and building upon the Credit Accumulation and Transfer Scheme (CATS) would be the preferable solution. This would ensure education which has the breadth and depth required for autonomous and accountable practice (unlike the example of an A&E NP curriculum given by Burgoyne (1992), which only lists the essential medical components) whilst also ensuring that the nurse received due credit for the work done in terms of CATS points contributing towards a degree. Essential technical skills could be included in such a package which, with the flexible modular approach now used in higher education, could be tailored to meet the individual's needs.

The second problem concerns an arbitrary list of criteria which exclude many patients from the NP's care, with no logical reasons or rationale given. This approach is found in other UK papers on the subject (Head, 1988; Burgoyne, 1992; Howie, 1992). Statements like: 'Walking patients presenting with minor injuries must be over the age of 12' are difficult to justify. What is meant by walking? Does that include capable of walking, but the ankle sprain is painful so the patient would rather sit in a wheelchair? Does limping count as walking? Why the age limit of 12? Why not 11 or 13? Children develop at many different rates; this arbitrary limit has no rationale. A significant number of patients come to A&E without injuries wanting advice, needing health education; why exclude these patients?

The NP according to Potter is excluded from treating any wound involving the cosmetic area of the face – why? Is this a sense of insecurity? Are we saying there is a greater risk of the NP treating the wound inappropriately and the patient consequently taking legal action because it is the face? Such a blanket ban is unprofessional and ritualistic as it is symptomatic of unthinking practice. Surely it is more sensible, and in line with the UKCC *Scope of Professional Practice*, to state that the NPs will treat any wound they feel capable of treating. Correct education will ensure that only appropriate wounds within the competence of the NP are treated by the NP, whilst more challenging and complex wounds are treated by the doctor. A facial wound can be a minor scratch that requires no treatment other than reassuring the patient and cleaning up or a single Steristrip (eminently suitable for the NP to deal with), through to some horrendous wound needing the attention of a plastic surgeon.

It would be unrealistic to expect doctors to agree to an NP system without guidelines for triage. The point is that minute detail is not necessary if the nurse is held accountable for only treating patients that s/he feels competent to treat. Agreed guidelines should have rationales explaining why some types of condition must be seen by a doctor rather than the NP. Clearly there have to be limits in A&E which need to be negotiated with medical staff. They should however be rational, justifiable and consistent with the UKCC *Scope of Professional Practice* guidelines which have now replaced the extended role of the nurse. Arbitrary and petty rules imposed either from other groups or by management are ritualistic and the antithesis of liberation nursing.

The account given by Head (1988) is an interesting first step in the direction of the A&E NP and reviews the experience of a 10-week trial. One of the limitations of the work has already been discussed – the arbitrary limits imposed on practice. A second limitation was the lack of education provided for the role. Instead, 5 years' A&E experience as a registered nurse was adjudged sufficient to undertake the duties of NP.

The NP saw 12% of all patients attending A&E during the trial period and dealt with around 4%; the remaining 8% were referred to casualty officers. In total, 1393 patients were seen by the NPs, of whom 271 (19%) were treated and discharged, 79 (6%) were advised and 142 (10%) were referred to their own GP. The remaining patients (65%) were sent to X-ray by the nurse and their treatment taken over by the medical staff. This caused problems with the Society of Radiographers, who did not approve of nurses authorizing X-rays and the health authority had to guarantee vicarious liability for the actions of the NP in requesting X-rays.

There was a systematic internal audit of treatment based upon a sample of 50 patients in which the auditor agreed with the action taken by the NP for 88% of the sample and felt that in the remaining 12% possible alternative treatments would have made little if any difference to outcomes. This is reassuring and highlights the potential of the NP. The report mentions a substantial degree of patient approval (91% said they were satisfied with treatment from the NP) when the Community Health Council (CHC) investigated the outcome of the trial, but does not elaborate upon sample size or response rate. This is an unfortunate weakness in evaluating the study.

A less satisfactory account of an NP trial comes from Howie (1992). In his unit it was decided that all registered nurses would become NPs and that training would be given by the medical staff. It is illogical to talk of NPs in one breath and in the next turn over their training to doctors! This shows a fundamental misunderstanding of the NP concept and demonstrates a failure to meet the most important criteria for NP development, i.e. that the role is fundamentally a nursing one. At least in Head's study, where significant experience was felt to be sufficient from an educational viewpoint, the nurses had learnt a great deal from other nurses.

The second major criticism of Howie's study, apart from the arbitrary limits imposed on practice, is the statement that: 'Nurses who have been trained, act as practitioners when they are available and a doctor is not'. There is clear evidence here that the nurse acts as a substitute doctor, not an NP. It is demoralizing to have staff constantly changing roles, being judged capable of taking on extra responsibility one minute but not the next. Any second level (formerly enrolled nurse) will recognize the effect this has on morale. Sadly, this approach fails to meet any of the criteria for NP or liberation nursing and merely relegates nurses to the role of part-time doctor's assistant.

The NP work in primary health care involved a great deal of health education and advice-giving. The literature on the NP in A&E has only referred to minor injuries. This is a wasted opportunity for, while minor injuries are undoubtedly a major component of NP work, the health-promotion side of nursing should not be overlooked.

Much has been written about 'inappropriate attenders' at A&E – patients with trivial injuries and conditions who could have gone to their GP, assuming they had one. There is, however, substantial research to demonstrate that the concept of inappropriate attendance is fundamentally flawed (Walsh 1990, 1993a, 1993b), for it is not the patient who is inappropriate but the service offered by the A&E department. Walsh has shown that patients make rational choices about attending A&E: the fact that their perceptions are different from medical and nursing staff does not make them inappropriate. Benner and Wrubel (1989) have argued the case for nurses to recognize what they call the 'situated meaning' of illness for a patient. In other words, a health problem has a meaning to the patient that depends upon the individual's situation, which is likely to be very different from that of the nurse or doctor. Neither is right or wrong, just different.

NPs could offer appropriate treatment and health education for many A&E patients if they also saw non-trauma cases, subject of course to agreed triage protocols. In the process they would be offering an alternative service for patients, fundamental to the concept of the NP, and also patient empowerment which is enhanced by choice. The NP would also further relieve the workload on medical staff who would then be free to concentrate on more seriously ill and injured patients.

The nurse practitioner and liberation nursing: a summary

In this chapter the concept of the NP has been examined and shown to contain great potential for liberating nursing. It is an idea that the profession should embrace and carry forward. The concept of nurses practising in an autonomous and accountable fashion is what matters rather than arguments about titles, and the challenge for the UKCC is whether it is prepared to support this concept. Does it see the characteristics of the NP outlined in this chapter as synonymous with a nurse operating at its 'advanced level' of practice?

Benner and Wrubel (1989) have pointed out that the practice of nursing can be frustrated by the writing of rigid rules that proscribe and limit nursing and criticize managers for getting in the way of expert nurses by insisting upon regulations that serve only to constrain rather than facilitate expert nursing practice. These authors point out that this bureaucratic approach to nursing may have its origins in high staff turnovers, as managers seek to limit the chance of error by writing rules and procedures for everything rather than trusting the professional accountability of the nurse. The casualization of the nursing workforce in the UK which is taking place in some areas as a cost-cutting measure may produce the same undesirable consequences. We have already seen that the natural and understandable caution of doctors involved in NP development is being translated in practice into arbitrary constraints upon nurses which have little logic and which will strangle the NP role.

The role of nursing education in preparing the NP is crucial. If nursing in the UK makes the mistake of thinking that only a low-level education is needed to function as an NP, the result will not be a practitioner of nursing excellence. Worse still, if education is handed over exclusively to doctors, the result will not even be a nurse. It is undeniable that significant areas of knowledge and certain skills need to be acquired by the NP which can be best taught by a doctor, but there is much else that lies within the domain of nursing and the social sciences.

Nurses could make claims to increased status and expertise by emphasizing and developing their highly specialized knowledge of science and technology rather than the caring dimension. Benner and Wrubel (1989) admit this possibility but urge nurses to recognize their scientific, biomedical knowledge for what it is – a tool, a means to an end, and that end of course is caring, which is the touchstone of nursing. In their view, to make scientific and technical biomedical knowledge the primary source of nursing's legitimacy assaults the inner logic of nursing practice. The reader is also reminded of Freire's warning that a characteristic of a subordinated group is to seek to imitate the culture of the dominant group, in this case medicine (Chapter 3).

Flexible modular programmes linked to higher education, earning CATS points and qualifications up to degree level (such as the ENB Higher Award) offer a very promising way forward in preparing the NP. This approach will allow the development of the necessary width and depth of expertise and knowledge whilst earning academic credit for doing so along the way. Real excellence develops in practice, however, and as Benner and Wrubel state (1989), the development of nursing knowledge will be greatly assisted by feedback from experts in clinical practice fuelling the educational process.

The development of the NP may not lead to liberation nursing if, even in independent practice, the nurse adheres to medical styles of patient interaction. A study by Taylor *et al.* (1989) compared the interactional styles of doctors and NPs with patients to three theoretical types of interaction. These were described as paternalistic (directive, instruction-giving), maternalistic (consequential, i.e. 'If you don't do this then this will be consequences...') and shared decision-making (concordance, mutually negotiated and agreed goals).

This study involved 127 video-taped consultations of 85 doctors (80 male, 5 female) and 42 NPs (39 female, 3 male) interviewing patients. A total of 906 attempts to influence decision-making were analysed. The following statistically significant results emerged:

- Doctors were more likely to use directive, instruction-giving methods of persuasion than NPs.
- Male NPs were more likely to use directive methods than female NPs (no difference was observed between male and female doctors, however).
- NPs were more likely to use consequential methods than doctors.
- Doctors used directive methods more than any other method.
- Both groups used concordance or shared decision-making strategies less than any other approach.

This study demonstrates that NPs approach attempts to influence patient decision-making differently from doctors. Paternalism is grounded in the premise that the person is justified in making the decision for the patient. The maternalistic approach has been described by Taylor (1985) as laying out the consequences of decisions for patients rather than discussing alternatives. This is seen as using the 'language of selfishness and responsibility to gain patient cooperation or acquiescence to decisions already made by the health care professional or family'. Empowerment of patients is concerned with shared decision-making, and in this study the NPs were as unlikely to use this approach as the doctors.

Styles of influencing decision-making need to be addressed in NP education in order to avoid falling into the traditional medical paternalistic style and to facilitate genuine joint decision-making with patients rather than the maternalistic style described here, which at times can seem like moral blackmail. Empowerment requires shared decision-making.

The development of the NP offers great potential for nursing, but it also may fall into the trap of becoming a ritualistic form of practice if nursing does not control the educational process for NPs, and if their role is circumscribed by a mass of arbitrary rules and regulations which deny the NP the chance to be innovative and creative whilst working within professional nursing guidelines. Doctor's assistants are not NPs!

Relationships with other professional groups and managers hold the key to development and nurses should scan the dramatically changing field of health care in the UK today and look for opportunities. Why should community NPs be tied to general practice? What is to stop nurses organizing in such a way as to sell their services as independent practitioners to the NHS, utilizing the internal market framework? Perhaps it is time for some daring and radical thinking?

Recommendations for good practice

NPs should

- Enhance patient services, offering new and alternative choices to services that are already available.
- Have a holistic, health-based view of patients.
- Have an education that is nursing-led, sensitive to local needs and which leads to degree-level qualifications.
- Have an identifiable theoretical framework within which they operate, e.g. the health belief model.
- Possess a large degree of autonomy.
- Recognize their accountability to the UKCC, the law (both civil and criminal), their employer and also themselves.
- Always remember they are a nurse, not a doctor's assistant.

References

Andrews S (1988) An expert in practice. *Nursing Times* **84**: 26, 31–32.
Barker P (1988) A genuine art. *Nursing Times* **84**: 36, 44–45.
Benner P (1984) *From Novice to Expert*. Menlo Park, Addison Wesley.

Benner P, Wrubel J (1989) *The Primacy of Caring*. Menlo Park, Addison Wesley.

Bowling A, Stilwell B (1988) *The Nurse in Family Practice*. London, Soutari.

Burgoyne S (1992) Emergency nurse practitioners. *Nursing Standard* 6: 27, 12.

Burke-Masters B (1988) Nurse practitioners in British general practice. In: Bowling A, Stilwell B (eds) *The Nurse in Family Practice*. London, Scutari.

Casey N (1993) PREP falters at first hurdle? *Nursing Standard* 7: 27, 3.

Castledine G (1982) *The Role and Function of Clinical Nurse Specialists*. University of Manchester MSc. thesis.

Covington C, Sellers P (1992) Implementation of a nurse practitioner staffed fast track. *Journal of Emergency Nursing* 18: 124–131.

DHSS (1986) *Nursing: A Focus for Care*. Report of the Community Nursing Review. London, HMSO.

Dimond B (1990) *Legal Aspects of Nursing*. London, Prentice Hall.

Freire P (1985) *The Politics of Education: Culture, Power and Liberation*. New York, Macmillan.

Head S (1988) Nurse practitioners: the new pioneers. *Nursing Times* 84: 26, 27–28.

Howie P (1992) Development of the nurse practitioner. *Nursing Standard* 6: 27, 10–11.

Huch M (1992) Nurse practitioners and physician's assistant, are they the same? *Nursing Science Quarterly* 5: 52–53.

Markham G (1988) Special cases. *Nursing Times* 84: 26, 29–30.

NHS Management Executive (1993) *Nursing in Primary Health Care: New World, New Opportunities*. London, HMSO.

Potter T (1990) A real way forward in A&E. *Professional Nurse* 5: 586–588.

Salisbury C, Tettersell M (1988) Comparison of the work of a nurse practitioner with that of a general practitioner. *Journal of the Royal College of General Practitioners* 38: 314–316.

Shuttleworth A (1991) A chance to accommodate high flyers. *Professional Nurse* 6: 488.

Slauenwhite C (1991) Independent nurse practitioners. *Canadian Nurse* 87: 24.

Stilwell B, Greenfield S, Drury M, Hull F (1987) A nurse practitioner in general practice: working style and pattern of consultations. *Journal of the Royal College of General Practitioners* 37: 154–157.

Stilwell B, Drury M, Greenfield S, Hull F (1988) A nurse practitioner in general practice: patient perceptions and expectations. *Journal of the Royal College of General Practitioners* 38: 503–505.

Taylor S (1985) Rights and responsibilities; nurse–patient relationships. *Image: The Journal of Nursing Scholarship* 17: 9–13.

Taylor S, Pickes J, Geden J (1989) Interactional styles of nurse practitioners and physicians regarding decision making. *Nursing Research* 38: 50–55.

UKCC (1993) *Community Education and Practice Proposals*. London, UKCC.

UKCC (1993) *Post-Registration Education and Practice Report*. London.

Ventura M (1988) Assessing the effectiveness of nurse practitioners. *Nursing Times* 84: 9, 50–51.

Walsh M (1990) Patient's choice, GP or A&E department. *Nursing Standard* 5: 10, 28–31.

Walsh M (1993a) Delaying attendance at A&E departments. *Nursing Standard* **7**: 33–35.
Walsh M (1993b) A&E or GP? How patients decide. *Nursing Standard* **7**: 36–38.

9 Care plans, process and models

Introduction

The nursing process, care plans and models of nursing have been advocated by many nurses as a means of moving nursing away from depersonalized, task-focused traditional styles of nursing towards an individualized, patient-centred philosophy of care. Primary nursing is another such initiative with a similar goal. It is now over a decade since the nursing process became widespread in the UK; nursing models followed a little later; now is therefore a good time to take stock of these cornerstones of current nursing theory.

The principles of liberation nursing which we believe might empower nurse and patient alike will be used as a framework for analysing the value of care plans, the nursing process and conceptual models of nursing. This exercise will be conducted utilizing the findings of experience and research which have been carried out in the last few years. The conventional wisdom that has been delivered under the banner of the nursing process may well be ready for serious challenge, as we shall see.

Do nurses know what the nursing process is?

An analysis of the nursing process has to start with this obvious question. Most readers will be familiar with the assertion that care should be planned on an individual basis, starting with assessment of the whole patient, from which problems both actual and potential are deduced. Realistic, patient-centred and measurable goals are set and the care to be implemented to achieve those goals is written out longhand before implementation. Evaluation of the effectiveness of care leads to reassessment and the process continues in this circular fashion.

That is the basic approach taken very early in nurse education. An old teaching adage should be recalled here, however – 'It's not what is taught that matters, but what is learnt'. The two may therefore be very different, so rather than assume that nurses understand the nursing process in the same way that tutors teach it, we need to start by looking at investigations into nurses' understanding of the nursing process and care-planning in the real clinical environment. The comment by Woolley (1990) that every nurse asked to define the nursing process will give a different answer might be overstating things a little, but contains a substantial element of truth.

The importance of clarifying exactly what nurses mean when they talk about the nursing process is underlined by Smith (1991), who suggested that there are two very different meanings in common usage. To some it is a philosophy which values and provides patient-centred rather than task-centred care; however, to others it is simply a method of organizing care. The similarity with the debate surrounding primary nursing is striking for, as we saw in Chapter 7, this too is seen in broad terms as a philosophy of individualized care by some, but only as a method of organizing care by others. The same comment might be applied to how nurses see the nurse practitioner role or quality assurance; is it part of the philosophy of individualized care or just another means of getting the work done? Nurses must clarify what they mean by terms before a meaningful discussion can occur.

It is interesting that nurses seem to see new concepts as either a philosophy of individualized care or more as a way of organizing the work. If this latter point of view prevails, the actual work that we do will remain unchanged and the potential benefits of individualized care will never be delivered because there will never be individualized care. Whatever new label is attached to care, tasks will still reign supreme.

It was the need to find out what nurses understood by the nursing process that led Sheehan (1991) to carry out an original and very interesting study which produced surprising results. The transition from task- to patient-centred care that the nursing process seeks to implement requires a fundamental conceptual shift. Sheehan wondered whether tutors and clinical nurses really had made that shift, or were they merely paying lip service to the ideals of patient-centred care and the nursing process?

A literature search led Sheehan to propose the following key words that are most closely associated with the nursing process: holistic, systematic, scientific, individualized and problem-solving. He set out to test this out by interviewing 40 nurses, 25 of whom were general and 15 who were from psychiatric and learning disability backgrounds. Of this sample, 29 were tutors and 11 were ward sisters. He used an open-question type of interview technique, focused around the subject's understanding of the nursing process. Responses were analysed by content and then a cluster analysis was undertaken; this produced clusters of nurses with similar responses on various topics. The sample fell into two large clusters and could be subdivided into five smaller clusters.

The first large group had 23 members who were predominantly general nurses (74%) and the more senior members of the sample, seven out of the eight senior tutors, fell in this cluster. They tended to see the nursing process only in terms of individualized as opposed to task-focused care. The second cluster had a grasp of more concepts associated with the nursing process, such as patient assessment, goal-setting and evaluation. Sheehan felt that the first group did not see the nursing process in its fullness; it was merely an alternative to another system of organizing care. The preponderance of senior tutorial staff with little recent clinical experience might explain this lack of awareness of the possibilities offered by individualized care-planning.

When the sample was divided into five smaller clusters, some very interesting detail began to emerge. Two clusters made little or no mention of evaluating care given and these were almost exclusively general nurses. Decision-making as a characteristic of the nursing process was conspicuous by its absence and those groups who said little about this crucial area also said little about implementation of care once planned. Problem-solving also figured infrequently in responses, whilst the concept of holism was largely absent, as was the notion of negotiating with patients over care. The notion that the work was scientific in approach was not mentioned at all, while many did not even mention a systematic style of care in discussing the nursing process.

These notions are all central to the concept of individualized care-planning using the nursing process format, yet very few nurses in this sample talked spontaneously about them when discussing what they meant by the nursing process. The fundamental validity of the work is supported by the fact that some nurses talked about some of the concepts, and all nurses talked about patient assessment and the importance of the individual: this at least gives the work some face validity as it assures us that the interviewer and nurses were, on the face of it, talking about the same thing!

There is a strong suspicion derived from this work that many of the nurses in question really had not internalized the concept of the nursing process as a means of delivering individualized patient care. One of the most frequently made points about the nursing process is that it is a rational problem-solving approach to planning care, yet many of these nurses seemed unable to talk of making decisions about care or solving problems. It is as if the assessment stage has become decoupled from the nursing process – everybody does that bit, but then the tendency appears to be to slip back to something else. Because the individual has been assessed, the assumption appears to be that the care is automatically individualized, when in practice there is little evidence from many of these nurses that it is, most worryingly shown by the lack of evaluation prevalent amongst general nurses.

Sheehan's work has shown that many of the central tenets of the nursing process, the conventional wisdom to be found in any textbook or college classroom, are perhaps only skin-deep in the real world. They have not been internalized by nurses in such a way that they flow naturally into conversation about the nursing process and care-planning. Sheehan's sample, of course, is small, and heavily weighted towards tutors, and the results not readily generalizable to the whole of nursing. Further, what nurses say and do may be two different things: practice may tell a different tale to that told in a research interview. Even when these allowances are made, it is clear that Sheehan's work is in urgent need of replication with follow-up studies – the central thrust of his findings remains disturbing. Is the nursing process really only skin-deep and what price empowering the patient, given the lack of awareness shown by these nurses of the importance of negotiation with the patient about care?

Nurses' understandings of the nursing process have also been investigated by Hurst *et al.* (1991). These authors set up a series of seven vignettes or patient profiles. These researchers were interested in letting nurses read about care in these vignettes and interviewing the subjects about the care described. The point of the study was to omit stages of the nursing process from different vignettes in order to see how this affected the way nurses talked about the care studies.

The results again raised the issue of how much nurses really have internalized the nursing process. When all reference to the planning stage was left out, only 25% of nurses commented on this omission; for the evaluation stage the figure was only 21% commenting on its omission. The suggestion is that care studies were accepted at face value when fundamental stages of care-planning were missed out with only around 20–25% of the sample raising the issue. Does this mean that most nurses did not notice crucial stages were missing, or, having noticed, did not feel it was sufficiently important to mention? An alternative explanation might be that they felt overawed by the research situation and so did not wish to dissent from what was placed in front of them.

The researchers interpret the study in terms of many nurses having an action focus which leads them to concentrate upon implementation at the expense of the more analytical stages such as evaluation and planning. It is a cause for concern, they continue, that many nurses did not comment upon what are widely held to be key stages in the nursing process.

If the researchers' results are accepted as valid rather than an artefact of the research situation, this raises several more concerns. To what extent is traditional nurse training to blame for an apparent lack of an analytical focus amongst these staff? If we are to proclaim the importance of the notion of reflective practice as a way of building and validating nursing knowledge, then the ability to evaluate and analyse care is crucial, yet these skills appear to take second place to a bias for doing, in the sample of qualified nurses and senior students studied here. The focus on practical care without thinking about what is being done and why stems from the well-known nursing tradition of following orders and of course explains much ritualistic care.

There is another possible radical explanation which has been rejected by these researchers. Nurses may not actually work in the logical staged way that the nursing process involves; consequently a study looking for evidence of these stages might find some nurses, particularly those with more experience, operating in a different way to that postulated by the nursing process. A lack of analytical skills and a bias for getting on with the job may well explain these findings, implying that many nurses have not really internalized the nursing process. We will return later to the more fundamental question of whether the nursing process is an accurate model of how nurses work in practice.

As a means of arriving at a reliable and valid measuring tool that could detect the nursing process in operation, Brooking (1989) undertook a major piece of methodologically rigorous research. This is recommended to all who would develop a measuring tool of their own as an example of how validity and reliability are established.

Brooking commented upon the lack of objective indicators which could determine whether a ward was using the nursing process: simply asking the staff is not an objective measure. As we have seen, concepts such as the nursing process mean different things to different people.

Brooking's final scale was developed from an initial list of 65 items identified in the literature which, after rigorous testing and checking, were reduced to a self-administered questionnaire taking 10 minutes to complete with a parallel observation schedule which could be used in any clinical area to complement the results of the questionnaire. Brooking admits though that the tool is very sensitive to documentation. This leads to the possibility that a ward may have individualized, planned care of the highest quality, but the score it obtains might not reflect the quality of care delivered because of its documentation. The nurse (or a patient) might ponder, which is more important? The significance of this work is the recognition that reliable and valid measures are required that allow us to recognize the nursing process when we see it. Such objectivity is crucial in any debate about its merits or otherwise: we have to be sure we are all discussing the same thing.

Why is the nursing process unpopular?

There is a widespread dislike of the nursing process in the UK, as a study of the letters pages in nursing journals over the years and eavesdropping on any staff-coffee-lounge gossip will attest. Why do staff resent what is claimed by nursing leaders and the statutory bodies as a crucial step in the professional development of nursing?

The first casualty when a ward gets busy is the written care plan, asserts Rundell (1991). He went on to suggest that nurses only pay lip service to the written care plan, with the result that documents are often ritualistic, outdated and at times dangerous, and bear little resemblance to the actual care given. If we are to be judged by our care plans in the future, Rundell wonders what people will make of the stilted, abbreviated clumsiness that masquerades as evidence of professional care. A care plan should be seen as a contract of care with the patient and not a bureaucratic chore. We need pride in our care plans, he concludes.

This *cri de cœur* will be recognized by many. Barnes, for example, writing in 1990, pointed out that care plans often bear little resemblance to the assessment they are supposed to be based upon. Nurses assess patients and discover a great deal of valuable, individual information but do not translate this into a plan of care. Instead, what appears is a ritualized plan written for the disease the patient is diagnosed as having, full of clichés and meaningless banalities. The result is that the standard of care bears no relationship to the written documentation. This is a key factor in examining the quality of care as various generic tools rely significantly upon written care plans. There is little evidence to correlate the quality of care plan and quality of care given.

Nurses are increasingly being asked to do more with less. The general impression in many areas over the last few years has been that staffing levels have at best failed to keep pace with the increasing demands upon nursing time brought about by factors such as increased patient throughput and dependency levels, the ageing hospital population and recent developments in medical technology. At worst we are seeing real cuts in registered nursing staff establishments and nursing redundancies. Against this back-drop, is the immensely time-consuming nature of the orthodox view of written, longhand care plans realistic? Not surprisingly, a nursing workforce who were originally very sceptical about the nursing process because of its top-down, coercive imposition (Walsh, 1991) are increasingly rejecting this approach to care, or just paying lip service to it. They have the right bits of paper available for audit if needed, but it is becoming more and more difficult for staff to carry out the nursing process in the conventional manner they have been taught.

What is the point therefore of care plans? Do they not represent an enormous waste of precious nursing time? Goodall (1988) asked nurses to consider that if the nursing process cannot be seen as the link between classroom theory and clinical care, then we should be honest and get rid of it, reverting back to task-centred care. Patients should be treated as diseases, collections of tasks to be performed, and not as individual people. Is that what we really want? He is critical of the pedantic longwinded process of writing out plans of care to which nobody pays any attention. As Manthey (1980) stated, 'No other piece of paper in a hospital system is as devoid of information as that entitled care plan'. Despite all the attention paid to assessment, the care plan that results is either of little value, or even if it has been conscientiously worked out, it is still often ignored.

It is little wonder that students, for example, resent such chores, as they are often the ones late off a shift as a result of having to fill in a care plan that is of questionable value. The whole exercise becomes a ritual. Tutors sometimes fail to realize the problems students face after being taught the nursing process in neat stages in college and then facing the real shock of wrestling with care plans in the clinical environment. Half-hour visits for a chat are not enough to appreciate fully the students' difficulties.

A lot of this criticism stems from the confusion in meaning that we highlighted earlier. The problem is that the nursing process has become obsessed with paperwork and the original intent behind the idea, that it should be a means of planning individualized patient care, has never really been internalized by staff. If the philosophy of individualized patient-centred care is thought of as a wood then it is a wood that we cannot see for the trees of ritualistic form-filling that the nursing process has come to represent. Ironically, if the nursing process continues consuming paper at its present rate, there will not be many trees of any sort left!

Research and the nursing process

Despite all the hopes and praise of nursing's leaders and academics, is there any research evidence to show that the nursing process has actually led to an improvement in care? As Chapter 6 demonstrated, measuring the quality of nursing care is an immensely difficult task and this is a problem that much research suffered from in the late 1970s and 1980s. In many projects methodological weaknesses have also been striking, such as reliability and validity issues, a lack of convincing evidence that the nursing process had been properly implemented, lack of equivalence between control and experimental groups when the experimental techniques were used and difficulties over timing. The net result has been a lack of any strong evidence to demonstrate that the nursing process improved care given.

It is worth briefly considering some of the more recent research papers that typify these difficulties. Richards and Lambert (1987), for example, investigated patient satisfaction with nursing care as a measure of the impact of implementing the nursing process. The reader is referred back to p. 116 for a discussion of the difficulties associated with this as a measure of quality. This study took place on a traditionally run psychiatric ward and involved questionnaires, patient interviews and numerical ratings of satisfaction.

The first problem with this study is that half the ward were said to be working traditionally at the same time as the other half of the ward operated the nursing process. It is difficult to see how staff could switch between the two halves without the style of working on one influencing their style on the other. Patients must have been similarly affected. A clear requirement of the experimental method is that experimental and control groups must be separate but equivalent. This second issue is not addressed in the research write-up; there is no evidence of testing to see if there was any significant difference between the two groups of patients in terms of age, gender, diagnosis, etc. There is no evidence of the questionnaire having been piloted or issues of reliability and validity discussed, let alone tested. The authors state that their questionnaire was testing in part the notion of the ward as a therapeutic community, which is not the same as assessing patient satisfaction, the stated aim. Validity is therefore questionable as the instrument is not measuring what it was supposed to be measuring.

The study found no difference between the views of the two groups of patients: the nursing process appeared to have made no difference. However, in view of this catalogue of methodological weaknesses, this study has little or no reliability or validity and the findings may be disregarded except to note that all the patients agreed in feeling that they could not influence care given in any way – hardly an empowering ward environment.

Another study which typifies the methodological problems of nursing-process researchers came from Hamrin and Lindmark (1990). This Swedish study looked at stroke patients and investigated the effects of introducing the nursing process on a ward by taking a series of measures on 107 patients prior to introduction in 1984 and on a further 173 patients after the introduction of the nursing process in 1985. The researchers reported no significant differences in patient groups or staffing during the two periods, establishing the equivalence of control and experimental groups lacking in the previous study. The introduction of the nursing process made no difference to the measures used to evaluate care.

They assessed the impact of the nursing process by measuring patient independence in activities of daily living, motor function and capacity, perceptual disturbance and carrying out a neurological assessment. This raises the issue of validity – to what extent are these physiologically based outcome measures a measure of the quality of nursing care given? Are they sensitive enough to detect any changes? A second problem concerned the statement that the researchers did not find that the registered nurses carried out the systematic care-planning. There is a silence about who did. However, if it was not registered nurses, is this an investigation of the nursing process? Brooking's methodological paper (1989) investigating just what is meant by the nursing process should be recalled to understand the importance of having a reliable and valid definition of the concept under investigation.

One final study will be examined and that is by Henderson and Southern (1990). Their starting point was that individualized care was an antidote to stereotyping of patients, particularly so with regard to groups such as the elderly or those with mental-health problems. This was an experimental design involving three groups of nurses and a vignette or patient profile. The control group filled in a questionnaire measuring attitudes towards the elderly while another group carried out a care-planning exercise based upon a real patient and then completed the questionnaire. The results showed that the experimental group had a significantly more positive attitude towards elderly care, leading the researchers to suggest that this was due to the intervening variable of carrying out an individual care-planning exercise.

In common with previous studies, there is no discussion of the reliability or validity of the questionnaire or of its piloting, whilst the equivalence of the experimental and control groups is not demonstrated. The difference in results could therefore be due to a difference in characteristics of the groups or an artefact of an unreliable or invalid questionnaire. Another possible explanation is that the control group were only dealing with abstract concepts in completing the questionnaire, whilst the experimental group had just had a concrete experience of care-planning. Perhaps the concrete nature of the care-planning experience altered their attitudes rather than the care-planning itself. We should remember that this was still a paper exercise and there is no evidence that these nurses would have behaved this way in practice. Finally, this is all based upon one patient profile only.

The nursing literature is replete with worthy attempts to show the value of the nursing process and individualized patient care which have foundered on the sort of methodological rocks outlined in the critiques of the three papers given above. Research in the area may be summed up as saying that it has failed to show that the nursing process makes any significant improvement in care. However, this infers more about the methodological difficulties encountered in researching nursing and the extreme difficulties in capturing and measuring such a complex and elusive entity as quality of care. As can be seen in Chapter 7, researchers in the field of primary nursing have had a similarly frustrating time. It is worth noting that Lawler (1991) sees a silver lining to this cloud, for in her view it has heightened our understanding of just how complex nursing is and reinforced the point that the most robust test of all is practice, and if after 15 years something is still not accepted in practice, like the nursing process, it has serious flaws.

One valuable aspect of Henderson and Southern's work is to put the spotlight on nurses' attitudes towards patients and the issue of stereotyping, the antithesis of individualized patient care. If a patient is seen as a 'typical' anything rather than a person, then individualized patient care is fatally undermined.

This point has been forcefully argued by Moss (1988), who reviewed the literature to find ample evidence of nurses stereotyping patients and expressing negative attitudes as a result, particularly in response to medical labels. Just some of the examples quoted include the effect of the label 'alcoholic', which has been shown to affect adversely nurses' perceptions of a patient, whilst female nurses have been shown to have more negative impressions of female compared to male patients, showing evidence of sex-role stereotypes. Moss argues that nurses' attitudes may have far more to do with determining nursing care than individualized care-planning, a point reinforced by Woolley (1990), who considers that the personal factors in the nurse–patient interaction are often overlooked. Prejudices and stereotypes get in the way of a detached, logical reasoning process, but as nurses are all human, they cannot be ignored.

Moss, for example, cites examples where, in the field of mental-handicap nursing, negative attitudes overruled the results of successful and popular client management and training programmes and led to their abandonment, whilst ritualistic toileting and other procedures which had no discernible beneficial effects were maintained.

The danger is that attitudes lead to self-fulfilling prophecies. If nurses treat patients in certain ways according to a set of fixed attitudes that conform to a stereotypical belief system, patients will tend to behave in that way eventually. Nursing care must be based upon the needs of the individual person, not a stereotype, yet as

Moss suggests, there is considerable evidence that nurses, while collecting individual information, still tend to carry out care for a *type* of patient based upon their own attitudes and beliefs, rather than the real individual. Whilst the research evidence in support of the nursing process is disappointing, we cannot go back to the traditional system of focusing only on tasks which have to be carried out for stereotypical types of patients, rather than real individuals.

Alternative approaches to care-planning

The model that students learn in college is of a rational stage-by-stage process in which an in-depth assessment is followed by carefully written out statements of patient-centred problems and goals; then nursing interventions are planned, carried out and of course evaluated. The process then begins again with reassessment.

Students are taught they should not use medical jargon or diagnostic language in writing nursing care plans. This results in hours of what Goodall (1988) has referred to as 'tautological frustration' as nurses struggle to avoid using medical language. As he suggests, if nurses could write down the medical diagnosis, this might save time spent reinventing the diagnostic wheel which could be more profitably used for care.

The rejection of medical labels was an understandable development in the 1970s and 1980s as nurses tried to get away from the medical model and establish nursing in its own right. However, there comes a point when Goodall suggests that common sense should be allowed to prevail, and incorporating simple medical diagnostic labels in care plans is perhaps one such area. The reader will remember that in our discussion of oppression in Chapter 3 the absorption of the language and values of the oppressors in a watered-down form into the subordinated culture was seen as a characteristic of one group dominating another. If we follow Goodall's suggestion, this might be argued as recognition of a *fait accompli*. Alternatively, in the long run if multidisciplinary care is to become a reality, perhaps some nursing language might cross professional boundaries moving in the opposite direction? There is of course the deeper point that the whole nursing process mimics medicine, so what is in a name anyway? This point will be explored later.

A more radical discussion that involves more than just changing the language of care plans is urgently needed, especially in view of the fact that the home of the nursing process, the USA, has now turned away from the orthodox care plan. The Joint Commission on Accreditation of Health Care Organizations (JCAHCO) is a powerful body in the USA. It sets standards which have to be met for accreditation as an approved health-care institute, one of which has been evidence of formally written nursing care plans. Brider (1991) reported that this requirement has largely been dropped in a recent review of accreditation standards and speculates that there will be a rapid demise of the traditional nursing care plan as a result.

This is not the same as the demise of the nursing process. Rather it is a decision that the correct place to document nursing care is in one set of notes with all other care received, including medical care. The new American requirements still insist upon documentary evidence of initial assessment, reassessment, patient care needs or nursing diagnosis, nursing care provided, outcomes of care and the ability of patients or significant others to manage care after discharge. The message is succintly summed up by the chair of the task force that produced this revision, June Werner, who is quoted by Brider as saying: 'We still have to show that a plan of care is in place, but it does not have to be that prototypical plan that students felt they had to write and which practising nurses weren't using'.

There is a green light for experimentation in this new requirement. As long as nurses can show care is planned on an individual basis and that it has the key six components mentioned above, they are no longer bound by the formalities of a care plan style that was originally designed as a teaching aid for students rather than a working document for experienced but busy registered nurses. Are British nurses prepared to liberate themselves from the tyranny of the conventional care plan and experiment with new ways of planning and documenting care? Brider poses the interesting question, should nurses be asked to write down for every single patient what they already know? This is a common complaint amongst nurses: care plans make them rewrite over and over again what they know. They feel they have to write a textbook every time they plan care.

The search should now be on for alternatives to the conventional care plan before it slips into the morass of ritualistic practice. Whilst few might mourn its passing in its present format, the danger is of throwing the baby out with the bathwater. Individualized patient-centred care, the philosophy that underpins care-planning and the nursing process, may disappear as well if the only alternative to the care plan is the task-focused bath book, bowel book, dressing book approach to care. Sadly, care-planning has been implemented in such a way by some nurses that it has become a modern-day ritual which has replaced the very rituals of the bath and bowel book that it was meant to abolish.

One alternative way of looking at care stems from evaluating the principles of care required for any given problem – they are fairly constant by definition, otherwise they would not be principles. Do nurses need to keep rewriting these principles in every care plan they write? As a registered nurse, an individual is assumed to know these principles and is held accountable for giving care based upon such principles. The art of nursing lies in adapting such general principles to individual patients' needs.

Considerations such as these give rise to the notion of the standardized care plan which is now gaining in popularity. The approach is based upon prewritten plans of care with interventions standardized upon common patient problems (Walsh, 1989, 1991) which can then be adapted to meet individual needs. The immediate objection, and it is a reasonable one, is that this leads to standardized care. All patients receive the same care regardless of individual needs. The danger is that this makes the assessment expertise of the experienced nurse redundant, together with individualized planning and care delivery skills.

In order to avoid this problem it is necessary to make sure that nurses fully appreciate the philosophy behind prewritten care plans and the requirement to address unique individual needs. If they are developed from amongst the ward team and grown from the bottom up to ensure a sense of ownership, they will probably have more chance of achieving this aim as they are seen as a ward staff's own solution to the problem of care-planning.

Developing core care plans or plans for the principles of care in this way can be a very empowering activity as all the care team can be involved, as also can patients and their families. The activity is very similar to standard-setting and it might be interesting to run the two projects in tandem. Reflection upon setting criteria which will demonstrate that standards of care have been achieved shows marked similarities with setting a principle-of-care goal (that the patient will state s/he is free of pain, for example). Quality standards and criteria can then be built into care-planning in an integrated way that meets the requirements of what in industrial quality jargon is known as zero deficit. This is explained by Muller and Funnell (1991) as building quality into a process rather than setting up a system whereby deficient products are inspected out. It is the process rather than the product that is subject to quality control. Health-care staff will be more familiar with this concept in the form of the prevention-is-better-than-cure maxim.

Building plans from principles of care draws upon the experience and expertise of all the ward team and as such may be expected to produce a stronger plan than any individual. The saving in time from not repeatedly writing out the obvious is potentially enormous. The key to success is in good assessment to identify where the problems lie that are amenable to a principles-of-care approach and what are the individual's unique problems that require a unique, customized plan of action. The use of a title such as a core care plan or a principles-of-care plan, instead of standard care plan, might avoid confusion with standard-setting and also avoid giving the wrong message about standardized care. Core care plans are being introduced as a means of conserving qualified nursing time in the care-planning exercise. Critics of this approach might argue that, rather than talk of core care planning, it would be more honest to say that the resources are not available for truly individualized care-planning. There are strongly held views on both sides of this debate.

In reviewing core care plans, Brider quotes Carpenito in describing the 'dinosaur system' of hand-written care plans and urging a move to a principles-of-care approach. What is the point, she asks, of identifying all manner of patient problems from an in-depth assessment if the nurse then does not have the time to do anything about most of them? Core care plans, however, which contain no evidence of addressing problems on an individual basis, must be seen as suggesting substandard care.

An alternative method of planning care involves nurses and doctors collaborating in planning a pathway that each patient is expected to follow. This critical pathway then maps out the normal trajectory of care that an individual should follow; hand-written charting records only the deviations from the expected pathway. Again, the analogy with standard-setting is striking as standards and criteria can be built into the critical pathway. Anything that promotes true collaboration between the different professional groups involved in patient care should be encouraged and the critical pathway approach could be extended beyond medical and nursing staff.

There is a danger however of this approach becoming very directive and devaluing the patient. It is perhaps more suitable for short-stay patients. Even so, the patients' view of their 'pathway' should be obtained and modification in light of the patients' wishes should be possible. This would also constitute an excellent information-giving opportunity and a chance to relieve a lot of patient anxieties about what will happen next. Brider reports that this approach has halved the amount of time nurses spend charting care in a study at St Luke's Hospital, Milwaukee.

Developments such as these are greatly facilitated by the spread of computers into the clinical environment as they are able to store the information needed to generate principles-of-care plans or critical pathway charts. Instead of writing an entire core care plan for a patient who has had a myocardial infarction, another for somebody who has had a cerebrovascular accident and yet another for an insulin-dependent diabetic patient admitted in a coma, computers allow a much more sensitive approach. Rather than one care plan for a 'standard patient', it is possible to build up a series of units consisting of principles of care for specific problems, which can then be assembled into a care plan for any individual, depending upon how the nurse assesses the patient. Such a plan still requires individual tailoring to the patient's needs. In addition to adapting computer-generated units of care, the nurse will still probably have to handcraft part of the care plan around unique problems. There will always be more individual problems than can ever be realistically identified and stored on a computer

The recording of nursing care for research into its effectiveness was cited as one of the many advantages of the nursing process. Unfortunately, the low quality of much of what is written and the dubious correlation that exists between written care plans and actual care means that this hope has remained unfulfilled. A computerized care-planning approach however reopens the possibility that nurses may be able to record care given, and its outcomes, accurately. The valuing of the clinical nurse and the knowledge that is contained within clinical practice has been urged as one of the keys to liberating nursing. The development of a database which allows us to investigate and demonstrate the impact of care upon outcomes would give nursing a golden opportunity to make such a breakthrough. Computer-based care-planning systems which valued the nurse's brain rather than hand-writing skills could make this achievable.

Before getting too carried away, however, with the possibilities offered by computers, it is instructive to look at some UK evaluations of what is currently available or possible. Standley (1992) has reported upon such an exercise, carried out by North-East Thames Regional Health Authority, which looked at software available to assist care-planning in the UK.

The first problem came with software that claimed to generate assessment packages. They were all felt to be much too preoccupied with the physical dimension of the individual and ignored the psychosocial aspects. They also involved duplication of effort for the nurse had to collect the information by hand and then type it all into a terminal. The next problem concerned keeping care plans updated on a computer as, unless the nurse had good typing skills, this would be even more time-consuming than the present system. In short, the evaluation exercise concluded that there are major problems with what is currently available. Perhaps these stem from trying to mimic with a computer the conventional approach to care-planning, and all the problems identified above. Time spent writing longhand is not saved by writing the same information at a keyboard unless the person has good typing skills.

If, however, the units-of-care approach is used and nurses can call up prewritten 'chunks' of a care plan and then adapt and assemble them to make a tailor-made plan of care, computers could then be seen as saving time. A very interesting account of just such an approach in the UK has been written by Yates (1992), who showed what could be done with a simple desktop personal computer on a 30-bed trauma ward. The ward team built up a total of approximately 200 commonly encountered patient problems and the principles of care required. They are now able to assemble a care plan utilizing whatever problems the patient assessment reveals. The staff are reported as feeling it is more detailed, much quicker and more legible than anything they had before. The scope for individualization remains, however.

Evaluation of the effectiveness of initiatives such as this is urgently required. The staff themselves reported that only having access to one terminal caused delays and the fact that the personal computer is not connected to the main hospital computer system means that the full potential of the system is not realized. Much information is lost which could be used within the rest of the hospital as a result. Quality assurance work is underway using the data stored on the computer for audit purposes. Imagine the power of such a system if standards of care are integrated into the chunks of care plan stored on the computer, therefore guaranteeing that every care plan will aim to meet agreed standards.

Standley (1992) points out the empowering potential of a computer-based approach to care-planning as the database of nursing care and its outcomes will be a powerful weapon to use when debates take place about the allocation of resources. Nurses may at last be able to show their worth and, in doing so, win control over resources which, apart from liberating the profession, will also allow us to invalidate the argument that nurses cannot be held accountable because they have no control over the allocation of resources for care.

It is important to return to an earlier theme however. There has to be evidence that the written care, be it computer-printed or painstakingly written longhand, actually translates into care given and that that care makes a real difference to patient outcomes. Audits of quality are still required.

The search for greater value for money in the NHS and the financial restraints under which we have to operate are increasingly leading nurses to have to care for patients who have not usually been on their ward. For example, patients with head injuries appear on surgical wards alongside women who have had gynaecological surgery. Nurses being called upon to care for patients with unfamiliar conditions could be greatly helped by the availability on a hospital-wide basis of a series of computerized principles-of-care plans, dealing with specific problems, which could be assembled into an individualized care plan.

Standards of care, because they were written into the individual units from which the plan is made up, can also be maintained across the whole hospital in this way. The elderly lady with a fractured neck of femur admitted to a general surgical ward, because the trauma ward has got beds closed, might receive better care as a result.

There are possible problems that may be encountered in building up a care plan from smaller subsections, the first of which concerns the possibility that any two subsections might be mutually exclusive. It is not uncommon for patients to be between the devil and the deep blue sea. A patient who has just had a myocardial infarction may initially require bed rest before beginning mobilization. The same patient may have a pressure sore or be at a high level of risk for developing a pressure sore. It is not difficult to see how two principles-based care plans may be at odds with each other, one advocating bed rest while the other aims at getting the patient out of bed. Unthinking implementation of the care plans for both problems could lead to absurdities. In practice, the experienced nurse compromises between the two differing requirements. This involves making a judgement about priorities and keeping the patient on bed rest, but turning 2-hourly. The nurse's brain will always be required to make these kind of judgements which is why, despite what some senior NHS managers think, patient care will always require professional nurses.

A second problem might be that the computer plans become out of date. It is essential that the nursing team are continually reviewing, in the light of current research findings and other information, the database on the computer. Care plans can become just as out of date and ritualized using this approach as they can in the traditional style.

Advocates of primary nursing might object to such an approach, but it is consistent with primary nursing principles. Individualized care can be delivered for which the nurse may be held professionally accountable, providing that assessment and reassessment are meticulously carried out, principles of care are adapted sensitively to the patient's needs and unique problems requiring unique solutions are recognized and acted upon accordingly.

If there is inadequate software to carry out the tasks that nurses require in planning care, then the whole computer approach to care-planning is an unproductive use of scarce nursing time. Time is wasted if nurses are not properly trained in the use of any system, however good it may be. A half study day is commonly the only preparation and is clearly insufficient. Nurses need to learn touch-typing skills as the painfully slow two-fingered typing that most nurses still use simply takes too long. If nurses are sitting at a keyboard long after the end of their shift, tapping patient data into a computer, then information technology can hardly be said to be improving nursing care. The whole resource management initiative is running into similar problems as the combination of inadequate software and lack of staff training in computer skills are leading to an unworkable mess.

Nurses who showed a willingness to change and accept the great information technology revolution heralded by the introduction of computers into clinical areas are now feeling demoralized as they spend large amounts of their own time or time which should be spent on patient care feeding the insatiable appetite for more and more data that seems to characterize computers. Other nurses query the large amounts of money being spent by some NHS trusts to ensure that every ward sister has a laptop computer at the same time as nurses are being made redundant and staffing levels reduced.

There is a fundamental problem remaining, which Standley (1992) pointed out – if nurses are not committed to individualized care-planning, no amount of computerized assistance will help. There needs to be a culture which approves of care-planning. How the nursing process was introduced could not have been better calculated to contradict all the principles of the management of change if people had tried. Cynics might argue that this was precisely the intent, thereby ensuring the failure of patient-centred care. Development of critical pathways or principles-of-care prewritten care plans will only succeed – along with any other nurse initiative to improve how care is planned and documented – if it is led by the staff who wish to explore such changes in an attempt to improve patient care. The repetition of these mistakes by half-baked implementation of information technology could prove a similar costly mistake. Computers could make a great contribution to care-planning but, as we have seen, they could also be an expensive disaster.

Nursing diagnosis and care-planning

Another related development in the USA which might impact upon care-planning is the development of nursing diagnoses. A nursing diagnosis is a standardized statement of a patient problem that attempts to take into account the whole person rather than just a part of the person, as a medical diagnosis does. Booth (1992) has advocated their introduction in the UK, stating that they are concise, precise, universally understood statements related to commonly occurring clusters of signs, symptoms and behaviours. Each diagnosis (there are approximately 90) is accompanied by related factors and defining characteristics which enable the nurse carrying out the patient assessment accurately to assign a series of nursing diagnoses to the patient. The familiar 'Patient Problem' column of a care plan is therefore replaced with a column headed 'Nursing Diagnosis'. The advantages claimed for this approach are that nurses are speaking a common language which should greatly improve communication and nurses can get rid of the vague generalities or cryptic shorthand that frequently pass for patient problem statements.

Are nursing diagnoses a useful way of speeding up care-planning? Turner (1991) has urged the development of care plans based around nursing diagnosis as a response to the problem of non-compliance with the requirement for care-planning by nurses which threatened accreditation under the former American standards. She found the two reasons given by nurses for not having care plans written was unfamiliarity with nursing diagnosis and lack of time. The response was a combination of in-service training and the development of care plans written for each nursing diagnosis which could be added to any patient's care plan after assessment, allowing the building up of a series of nursing interventions aimed at the principal patient problems. The need to individualize these plans is acknowledged.

The idea is very similar to that described earlier when we discussed principles of care – except for the crucial difference that these plans are built around nursing diagnoses. For this to be a valid approach to care – and it is regrettable this paper gives no report of staff evaluation of the change – the nursing diagnoses must themselves be valid and easily recognized by staff. The alternative is that staff will assess and implement the wrong care plan because of confusion over which nursing diagnosis to use.

Nursing diagnoses might therefore speed up care-plan writing and lead to clearer statements of patient problems that should be universally understood. However, they also have drawbacks, which have been the subject of a trenchant critique by Webb (1992). Starting with the American definition of a nursing diagnosis as a standard taxonomy of diagnostic labels that convey the same meaning to all nurses, Webb first pointed out that the large majority are only concerned with physical factors at the expense of the psychosocial domains of care, whilst the wording is frequently tortuous and obscure in the extreme. The element of standardization also threatens individualized care. These two criticisms alone make their use in the mental-health areas of nursing extremely problematical.

Diagnoses tend to be constructed in three parts – a patient quality or characteristic; a statement about its quantity (excess, deficit, lack, alteration in, etc.) and then finally whether the problem is actual or potential. The result is at times difficult to comprehend and, as

Webb points out, creates a real barrier to involving patients in their care.

Equally worrying for Webb is what is missing. There are no diagnostic statements, for example, about common problems such as pressure sores, nausea or itching whilst the only feeling or sensation a patient is allowed to have is pain. To Webb they are 'a rigid list of problems written in a bizarre format' and the strong medical links which are apparent from the physiological bias (apart from the word 'diagnosis' itself) represents a backwards step which could undo much of what has been achieved in the last few years.

An even more scathing attack upon nursing diagnosis is mounted by Lawler (1991). She argues first from a philosophical perspective that they represent the imposition of an inappropriate positivist, reductionist scientific culture upon nursing which espouses a more holistic approach to human understanding. Her second major criticism is that they were developed in the USA as a result of an economic necessity that had nothing to do with care at all. The economics of the American health-care system made it crucial to cost and account for nursing care, hence nursing diagnoses are a convenient way of breaking down these costs per patient. Lawler argues that turning nursing into a quantifiable science simply to keep the accountants happy is not how we should proceed. She raises a series of other objections concerning the validity of nursing diagnoses, for example, whether there is any demonstrable link between them and nursing care. In other words, do they actually make any difference to the care given?

This latter point has been developed by Mitchell (1991) in a powerful critique of nursing diagnosis. The point of medical diagnosis is to classify conditions in order to facilitate prediction and control. Nurses who carried out the development work on nursing diagnosis followed in this tradition, deriving their diagnoses according to Mitchell, not from theoretical conceptions about humans, health and ways of supporting and nurturing but from the traditional medical worldview. Freire's critique (1985) springs to mind – subordinated groups tend to take on the language, concepts and values of the oppressor in a watered-down form at the expense of their own culture. Mitchell is arguing that nurses have done precisely this with diagnoses and is therefore opposed to their use on the grounds that they exist to allow nurses to classify, predict and control patient behaviour, which is the antithesis of her supportive, patient-centred view. Nurses are taking away the patients' independence and sense of control over their health by the use of nursing diagnosis.

A further critique Mitchell makes is that to make diagnoses in this way requires an objective, reductionist perspective which is the opposite of the sort of nursing we should be aiming for. Nursing should be an activity which is supporting the integrative health processes of human beings. Mitchell urges nurses to focus on health-as-process and quality of life as defined by the individual (a very empowering perspective) rather than the reductionistic, problem-centred approach of medical science. This latter phrase sounds very similar to descriptions of the nursing process and opens up this central tenet of current nursing to serious question. As we shall shortly see, there is a powerful critique unfolding which may mean that the nursing process as we now know it may no longer be considered appropriate for experienced nurses.

In the next section, the role of nursing models will be reviewed in the delivery of care. It is reasonable to ask whether nursing models are consistent with nursing diagnosis, as they are the two most recent major theoretical developments in North America. If the diagnostic labels developed in the nursing diagnostic taxonomy cannot be generalized across a range of nursing models, then the only alternative for a diagnosis-based practice is to develop a set of diagnoses for each model. As there are at least a dozen mainstream models, and currently approximately 90 diagnoses which have been arrived at without reference to any model, the result might be a thousand or more nursing diagnoses to be used in documenting care. This is not a realistic way of proceeding!

An initial investigation into the fit between nursing diagnoses and one nursing model has been carried out by Jenny (1991). She utilized a sample of 130 registered nurses with a mean of 14 years' nursing experience, who were enrolled in a baccalaureate completion course. They had all studied Orem's self-care model (Orem, 1990) and also nursing diagnosis as part of the course. She asked the staff to consider Orem's model with its 16 categories of self-care deficit which make up the framework for patient assessment (Walsh, 1991) and to assign a list of 80 nursing diagnoses amongst these 16 categories.

If nursing diagnoses are valid measures of patient problems within this relatively widely used and easily understood model, there should be a high degree of agreement about which diagnosis fits under which self-care deficit heading. Unfortunately, this was not the case in practice as these experienced nursing staff found it very difficult to match the two concepts. The eight universal self-care deficits attracted between 20 and 39 nursing diagnoses each, while the remaining developmental and health deviancy self-care deficits had between one and 18 diagnoses each. These latter deficits not only attracted a range of diagnoses, but the numbers of nurses assigning any one diagnosis to a self-care category were low – typically less than a third of the sample.

This study suggests that this large sample of experienced nurses found it very difficult to match up nursing diagnoses and the Orem self-care nursing model. This suggests that there is a major validity problem with these two theoretical constructs. As the Orem model is one of the easiest to understand, it suggests that some of the more esoteric nursing models might produce even bigger discrepancies when tested against the nursing diagnosis framework. If Orem's model is a valid view of nursing care, this suggests that the current menu of nursing diagnoses lacks validity and needs rewriting for use with Orem's model and similarly with other models. Alternatively, it is Orem's model that has the validity problem and any other model that cannot demonstrate substantial agreement with the nursing diagnosis framework. This represents a major theoretical problem which nurses who wish to use these two concepts together must resolve. Nursing models and nursing diagnoses cannot develop in parallel, each pretending the other does not exist, as the existence of one challenges the validity of the other.

Any move towards introducing nursing diagnoses in the UK therefore faces an uphill task in view of the sort of arguments deployed above. It is certainly difficult to see how they may act to empower the patient, especially given the impenetrable language in which they are couched. It could be argued that they also devalue the clinical nurse's expertise in assessing the individual patient's problems by reducing his/her expertise to a collection of standardized and tortuous phrases. The national imposition of such a system also takes away any sense of local ownership which we strongly argue is essential for any change to work. Care plans built up from prewritten, principle-focused units are open to the charge that they remove individualization. But they can be locally written and owned, couched in language that everybody understands and sensitive to local needs. The freedom to amend and individualize such units according to the patient's needs is the best guarantee against loss of individuality. This flexibility is lacking in nursing diagnoses however: they must be identical everywhere, by definition. Nursing diagnoses, in conclusion, are best left on the other side of the Atlantic.

Models of nursing

Much has been written about conceptual models of nursing in recent years, ranging from outright rejection as just another North American import we can do without, through to total and slavish acceptance of a one-model-only approach. Neither position is very helpful (Walsh, 1991).

The basic aim of those responsible for producing models is to set out an ideal representation of one way of nursing, based around the interacting concepts of patient, environment, health and nursing. They are best seen as a guide to care which nurses can adopt and adapt to suit the patients cared for. The total acceptance of one model followed by a managerial edict to the effect that all patients will be cared for using this model only is unprofessional, ritualistic and, unfortunately, not uncommon, especially where the Roper model is concerned in the UK.

A weakness with many nursing models is that they suffer from a lack of obvious derivation from, and clear linkage to, the clinical practice they seek to guide. Fawcett (1992) acknowledges this problem and urges the need for a circular linkage between models and practice. As a model is tried in practice, staff should be reflecting upon its strengths and weaknesses, changing and adapting the model, perhaps grafting on sections of another model if it is philosophically consistent. In this way the model is dynamic and changing in response to real experience (Walsh, 1991).

The proponents of nursing models point out that nursing must have a starting point to guide practice as, if practice alone were the starting point for nursing knowledge, then nursing would be limited to first aid and disaster relief (Donaldson and Crowley, 1978). There is a tension here between the ideas of Schon (1983), which can be interpreted as emphasizing the supremacy of practice-derived knowledge whilst attaching much less importance to theory, and the proponents of nursing models who argue that we have to start somewhere. To some extent it is a circular process as practice and model each feed back into each other. If the circle is entered in one region it looks as though practice is fuelling theory, but enter the circle at another point and theory appears to be guiding practice. In a sense then both views are valid.

Of great value is the observation by Fawcett (1992) that a conceptual model should never be seen as ideology that cannot be altered. That way lies the road to ritualization. Jones (1989) has argued, for example, that models were devised to move nursing away from task-centred and ritualistic care towards more thoughtful practice: elevating them to the status of ideology will achieve the opposite effect from that intended. Models must be sensitive to practice and in this way reflection in action and reflection on action can both be brought to bear upon model development.

Not all models, however, translate into clinical practice. Nevin-Haas (1992) sounded a clear warning to theorists by pointing out that some, such as Rogers' model, are too abstract to have any real meaning while others, such as that of Neumann, are far too general and broad to give any real guidance to nurses. Nevin-Haas observes that nurses in practice must tell theoreticians when they are producing ideas that are incompatible with practice. This view of course might be criticized for propagating the theory–practice gap that many writers such as Schon and Benner wish to close by integrating theory and practice as one activity, rather than seeing theorists sitting apart in academic ivory towers.

If nursing care takes place as a result of nurses working with a linear, problem-solving methodology known as the nursing process (more expert nurses work in a more complex, Gestalt way, as we shall see in the next section), how do nursing models feed into these methods of working? It has been argued by Walsh (1991) that a model underpins the delivery of care via the nursing process and can only be fully implemented within a primary nursing system. It gives structure to the assessment and guides the nurse away from irrelevant areas; it also guides the way problems are understood and goals are set. It should also influence how interventions are carried out and evaluated. If the care delivered is identical, regardless of the model used, then either models are meaningless or a particular model has not been implemented. Model-guided care can therefore be delivered by the nursing process and the model can help shape the care delivered in this way.

The more experienced practitioner may not be following such a clear linear problem-solving process (Benner, 1984). Conceptual models, however, may still help shape care, although in a less explicit fashion. It is the philosophy behind the model that is more important, rather than the specific assessment headings which in their turn lead to problem identification and care-planning. The experienced nurse can choose which is the better approach to take from amongst the various philosophies on offer and vary and alter care in the light of experience and judgement. The blanket imposition of one specific nursing model is therefore fundamentally disempowering as it removes from the expert nurse the freedom to care in the way that s/he feels best suits any individual patient's needs. It also presupposes that all client groups' needs can be met by a single nursing model. The fact that imposed models are not home-grown products removes the sense of ownership that is so important and makes the introduction of a model in such a way yet another top-down management-led coercive change that, as we have seen, is unlikely to achieve staff acceptance. Chapter 11 demonstrates another way to approach the problem which did succeed; the staff developed their own model of care by reflection upon experience.

However, if a model is home-grown – developed by staff to reflect the values of care they believe in – then it is potentially very empowering for staff. Such a model can build in the patient's point of view and require his or her involvement, thereby empowering the patient as well as the staff. If the home-grown model is made broad and flexible enough, the freedom of professional judgement that is required for expert practice may be preserved. However, there is a fine balancing act involved, for the model must also give sufficient guidance to allow less experienced staff to see the structure it gives, within a care planning format, which they may find necessary for care.

Nursing models have the potential to be empowering if they are used in one of two ways. Existing models can be adapted by staff, in the light of real experience, to suit the needs of patients, or staff can develop their own model of care using a collaborative bottom-up approach. In either situation there is great potential to empower patients by involving them fully in the development of the model(s). The clinical nurse is valued in this way as critical reflection upon practice guides the development of nursing knowledge. Such an approach allows a model to influence how expert nurses carry out care on a broad philosophical level, whilst allowing junior staff to make sense of care by giving structure and clear purpose to care-planning. This approach allows nursing to develop practice that is grounded in the values and beliefs of nursing, rather than the imposed values of a dominant society such as medicine. It is therefore potentially very liberating.

The alternative approach should be recognized as dangerous. Imposition of single, narrow nursing models and their rigid interpretation, reinforced by nursing process documentation, is a serious threat to the freedom of expert nurses and should be resisted at all costs. Nurse educationalists have in some instances known to the authors suggested the removal of students if a single hospital-wide model was not adopted. That is the antithesis of education and it is also insulting to the intellect of students to suggest that being exposed to alternative approaches to care might so confuse them as to render invalid the whole educational experience a hospital could offer. Nursing will never be liberated if it is constrained by slavish obedience to literal interpretations of single narrow models which are accepted as ideology and which are isolated from feedback from the real world.

References

Barnes B (1990) When will we get it right? *Nursing Times* **86**: 4, 64.

Booth B (1992) Nursing diagnosis; one step forward. *Nursing Times* **88**: 7, 32–33.

Brider P (1991) Who killed the nursing care plan? *American Journal of Nursing* **91**: 34–38.

Brooking J (1989) A scale to measure the use of the nursing process. *Nursing Times* **85**: 15, 44–49.

Donaldson S, Crowley D (1978) The discipline of nursing. *Nursing Outlook* **26**: 113–120.

Fawcett J (1992) Conceptual models in nursing practice; the reciprocal relationship. *Journal of Advanced Nursing* **17**: 224–226.

Freire P (1985) The Politics of Education: Culture, power and liberation. New York, Macmillan.

Goodall C (1988) How should we teach the nursing process? *Nursing Times* **84**: 48, 47–49.

Hamrin B, Lindmark B (1990) The effect of systematic care planning after acute stroke in general hospital medical wards. *Journal of Advanced Nursing* **15**: 1146–1153.

Henderson P, Southern D (1990) Making care plans. *Nursing Times* **86**: 4, 33–35.

Hurst K, Dean A, Trickey S (1991) The recognition and non-recognition of problem solving stages in nursing practice. *Journal of Advanced Nursing* **16**: 1444–1455.

Jenny J (1991) Self care deficit theory and nursing diagnosis: a test of conceptual fit. *Journal of Nursing Education* **30**: 227–232.

Jones S (1989) Is unity possible? *Nursing Standard* **3**: 1, 22–23.

Lawler J (1991) In search of an Australian identity. In: Gray G, Pratt R (eds) *Towards a Discipline of Nursing*. Edinburgh, Churchill Livingstone.

Manthey M (1980) *The Practice of Primary Nursing*. Oxford, Blackwell Scientific.

Mitchell G (1991) Diagnosis: clarifying or obscuring the nature of nursing. *Nursing Science Quarterly* 4: 52.

Muller D, Funnell P (1991) *Delivering Quality in Vocational Education*. London, Kogan Page.

Nevin-Haas (1992) Checking the fit; nursing models, are we buying or just looking? *Canadian Nurse* 88: 33–34.

Orem D (1990) *Nursing: Concepts of practice* (4th edn). New York, McGraw-Hill.

Richards D, Lambert P (1987) The nursing process: the effect on patient's satisfaction with nursing care. *Journal of Advanced Nursing* 12: 559–562.

Rundell S (1991) Care about care plans. *Nursing Times* 87: 16, 32.

Schon D (1983) *The Reflective Practitioner*. New York, Basic Books.

Sheehan J (1991) Conceptions of the nursing process amongst teachers and clinical nurses. *Journal of Advanced Nursing* 16: 333–342.

Standley M (1992) Systems of care: computerised care planning. *Nursing Times* 88: 6, 53–55.

Turner S (1991) Nursing process, nursing diagnosis and care plans in a clinical setting. *Journal of Nursing Staff Development* 7: 239–243.

Walsh M (1989) *A&E Nursing: A New Approach*. Oxford, Butterworth-Heinemann.

Walsh M (1991) *Nursing Models in Clinical Practice; The Way Forward*. London, Baillière Tindall.

Webb C (1992) Nursing diagnosis; two steps back. *Nursing Times* 88: 7, 33–34.

Woolley N (1990) Nursing diagnosis; exploring the factors which may influence the reasoning process. *Journal of Advanced Nursing* 110–117.

Yates L (1992) Planning on a PC. *Nursing Times* 88: 23, 62–64.

10 *The nursing process: time for a change?*

In the preceding chapter we saw that many experienced nurses are unconvinced of the value of the nursing process and at best only pay lip service to it. On the research front, there is a lack of any evidence to support its use whilst in the USA, formally written care plans are no longer a requirement for accreditation. Individualized patient care remains the goal of most nurses, however, so is there an explanation for what has gone wrong and why basically the nursing process appears to have failed?

It is time to go back to beginnings. The nursing process is essentially a linear model. The nurse starts at point A, assessment, moves forward to point B where problems are identified, then on to set goals and on again to write out interventions. The nurse should then carry out these interventions before finally taking stock of the situation and evaluating their effectiveness. The nurse moves in a steady straight line, always in the same direction, stage by stage, hence the term 'linear model'. But does this methodical plodding

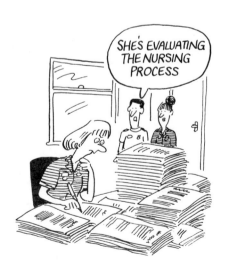

bear any resemblance to the way people work in the real world? Herein lies the crux of the issue.

This description of the nursing process corresponds well with one of the main decision-making models which is known as the stage model. Hurst *et al.* (1991) have reviewed this model and show that most accounts talk of problem identification, data-gathering, planning of actions, selection and implementation of strategies and evaluation of success. As they point out, this is very similar to the theory of the nursing process.

Hurst *et al.* however are very critical of the reality of the nursing process. In their view the literature demonstrates that nurses frequently fail to recognize problems, forget them, oversimplify or omit them, even when identified. Problem identification is taken as more than noting the existence of a problem: the nurse should also examine how it relates to others and look for possible causes. Failure to state clear and realistic goals will lead to a planning failure whilst the care implemented rarely resembles the plan acccording to these authors. Evaluation, they suggest, is the most important but least understood and effectively carried out stage of the nursing process. This analysis leads the authors to question the validity of the nursing process as a model for the way in which experienced nurses work in practice, despite what is taught in college to students.

In view of this failure, do we return to the task-focused ritualistic approach or perhaps we should be looking elsewhere for ideas about how nurses think and behave in clinical situations? A discipline which has spent over a century trying to describe and understand the way people think and behave is of course psychology. The early years of this century were marked by the work of people like Watson, Skinner and Thorndike who are associated with the behaviourist school of psychology. They aimed to make psychology a science and wished to deal in facts, causes and effects: they wanted to show that this stimulus leads to that behaviour in a logical and linear fashion. This has echoes of the linear, scientific nursing process approach.

However there was another school of psychologists who felt this was all too simplistic and in 1912 Wertheimer announced a new way of thinking about psychology – Gestalt theory. Gestalt means configuration in German, and these workers were much more interested in how human beings saw and perceived whole situations and the meanings attached to them. This led to a great deal of work looking at how humans learnt, set about solving problems and remembering things from the point of view of situations and the meanings and perceptions of those situations. Thinking was introduced instead of simple stimulus–response linkages and out of Gestalt psychology grew what in modern times has become known as cognitive psychology, whilst behaviourism has declined in importance. To students of Gestalt psychology, humans have the ability to perceive whole situations at once and decide what to do accordingly.

With that thought in mind, it is necessary to turn to the work of Benner (1984), who clearly showed that this is precisely how expert nurses function. The development of an expert nurse follows a path that after starting out as a novice depends upon rule-governed behaviour through the stage of advanced learner to competency. The advanced learner is always responding to situations rather than being in charge of them, in a sense analogous with the stimulus–response behaviourist picture. By the time the nurse has achieved competency s/he is following plans carefully and, as Benner states, 'The conscious deliberate planning that is characteristic of this skill level helps achieve efficiency and organisation'. However, as the nurse becomes proficient, according to Benner, s/he sees and understands situations as wholes because there is understanding of the long term and a wealth of experience has been accumulated to draw upon. The expert nurse has an almost intuitive grasp of the situation and seems to know naturally what to do without any thought.

It is worth entering a word of caution here. It is easy to get expert and experienced confused. It does not follow that an experienced nurse will be an expert unless learning has taken place along the way. A nurse may function by following orders and as a result of a ritualistic ward climate, lack of stimulation and other factors, may not necessarily progress beyond the rule-bound competent practitioner. That progression depends crucially upon critical reflection on practice.

The nursing process approach therefore seems appropriate to enable students to learn and make sense of nursing. The origins of the nursing process are indeed as an educational tool which was transposed into the clinical environment. In moving from student to newly qualified status, the nurse perhaps still needs the discipline of logic and order that the nursing process imposes in order to take responsibility for care that can be carried out safely. After a while, however, it becomes redundant.

Basic textbooks introduce students to the nursing process as a logical problem-solving approach to care-planning. It is worth pausing a moment to consider the language employed to do this and the less obvious hidden messages that are transmitted in basic textbooks. Critical social theory suggests that language is a key element in power (Habermas, 1976); consequently it is essential to think of how textbooks introduce students to this central plank of modern nursing – the nursing process.

Is language neutral or do distortions in communication help to maintain power by eliminating some concepts from discussion in favour of others? Habermas argues that language is a means to obtain power for when communication is restricted, social power leads to domination. The oppressed group cannot argue about something they do not know about, nor can they construct alternative approaches to problems if they are given only one conventional view of wisdom. Are nursing textbooks guilty of this charge by presenting only a conventional scientific view of the world and alongside it, the nursing process as the only way to carry out nursing care?

An interesting analysis of the language used in four North American textbooks to introduce the nursing process has been carried out by Hiraki (1992) and it is her conclusion that these books show a belief that the acceptance of nursing's professional status depends upon the adoption of scientific methodology. The nursing process is presented as a neutral problem-solving approach, removed from the context in which it occurs. Taking nursing process out of context in this way, according to Hiraki, removes the nurse from the need to question the social, environmental or political factors involved in the caring situation; all that matters is applying the process to the patient. Textbooks support the view that science is a neutral authority guaranteeing truth and excluding sociopolitical issues from debate in the health arena.

Is there evidence to support this assertion? Textbooks present an imitation of medical decision-making as the correct way of planning care for all nurses. This reinforces the dominance of the scientific model and of medicine. Nursing imitates and remains dominated by medicine, a thesis we have explored earlier in the light of Freire's critique (1985). Texts that present the student with an ideal way of planning care according to the nursing process do the student few favours when the real social world of a busy clinical area is encountered where nurses do not follow the textbook ideal. There is a tendency for the nursing process to disallow due recognition of the social factors involved in health as, according to the stylized way of presentation, there is little the nurse can do. Issues of deprivation, poverty and inequality are therefore excluded from nursing's agenda, despite their major effects on health.

There would appear to be a case to answer in response to Hiraki's charge concerning North American textbooks. Can we be sure that the approach taken to the nursing process in the UK absolves us of similar accusations, i.e. the language of the text in discussing the process acts as a form of control?

Hiraki is also critical of the way texts promote objectivity and the nursing process. She firstly questions what evidence there is to show that objectivity enhances nursing care and goes on to argue that objectivity in the application of the nursing process distances the nurse from the patient. There is a balance required between being too close to a patient and too remote. Primary nursing will, for example, bring a nurse much closer to a patient and therefore act in opposition to this distancing tendency. This may well set up tensions and strains that the nurse will have to recognize and work hard to resolve with colleagues. Hiraki interprets some US texts in encouraging this objectivity as actually giving the nurse substantial powers of coercion over the patient, especially in relation to value clarification.

If the nurse is assumed to be objective and scientifically neutral, then value clarification argues that the value systems of the patient are the ones that must be examined as the source of problems. The implicit argument seems to run along the lines that nursing is the yardstick against which patient values must be measured and changed accordingly to promote health. This is the very opposite of empowering patients.

In the preceding chapter evidence was presented that the nursing process amongst many UK nurses is only skin-deep – it has not been internalized. In view of the philosophical criticisms levelled against the nursing process in this discussion, it is perhaps as well that experienced nurses do not seem to be operating with the full (US) textbook model!

There is evidence therefore that a nursing process approach is of value in helping students learn and newly qualified staff nurses function. It is however open to charges that the concepts and language used in many texts may lead to the nursing process disempowering patients and also of being used as a means of controlling nurses. The nursing process as taught is inflexible, and leaves the experienced nurse trapped in a system of working that s/he may outgrow. The development of experiential learning and critical reflective practice may allow the nurse to grow into a Gestalt approach to patients and their problems. However, a lot of 'unlearning' of basic texts and rejection of conventional wisdom is required. The experienced nurse who makes this transition can see what needs to be done from a rapid assessment of the whole situation, without the reductionist and fragmented approach of the nursing process getting in the way. The experienced nurse no longer has a ball and chain around the ankle.

The connection between this total view of the patient and Gestalt theory was made in 1983 by Pyles and Stern, who coined the phrase 'nursing Gestalt'. They considered this consisted of a mixture of linking past experiences to gut feelings and present situational cues before deciding how to act. Some might call this intuition; others, such as Benner, define it as expert practice.

Intuitive judgement is something that many nurses will recognize. Benner and Tanner (1987) consider that there are six components which go to make up this nursing Gestalt. They are pattern recognition, similarity recognition, common-sense understanding, skilled know-how, recognition of prominent characteristics and deliberative rationality. Many of these characteristics develop from experience but experience alone is not enough. There must be learning taking place from the experience gained, which in turn involves reflection upon what is happening while it is happening and subsequently after it has happened. This critical reflective process is the core of Schon's (1983) argument about how practitioners learn to be experts (p. 52) and links with the ideas of Benner concerning the way nurses develop into expert practitioners.

Benner and Tanner have a place for the rational, linear, problem-solving approach, but argue it is not enough to explain how expert nurses function. It is a model that fits the student and newly qualified nurse, but not the expert.

In working with patients on a daily basis to optimize the shifting frontline that represents health, nurses make use of intuition and common sense, yet they shy away from talking of intuition, especially with the recent emphasis on the scientific paradigm.

Rew and Barrow (1989), for example, could find only one article title with the word 'intuition' contained in it in reviewing all copies of the *American Journal of Nursing* from 1900 to 1985. They also report that related concepts such as empathy, instinct and insight have occurred frequently and consistently throughout that period. It is as though nurses were afraid to use the word intuition in front of doctors, especially in light of the sex-role stereotyping that portrays this in a slightly derogatory manner as 'women's talk'. Rew and Barrow cite several research studies that reveal the importance of intuition in nursing (e.g. Schraeder and Fischer, 1987; Rew, 1988) and which also reveal the way nurses feel almost embarrassed to use the word because of hostile reactions from doctors.

The medical way of working is traditionally locked into the positivist, scientific method that has no place for an alternative approach incorporating such an unscientific concept which nurses refer to as 'intuition'. This ability to see the whole situation at once rather than in a fragmented linear way has an honourable lineage, for as we have seen, it played a crucial role in the development of psychology when expressed as Gestalt.

Rew and Barrow echo this critique of the nursing process when they look at the implications of nursing diagnosis. As a diagnosis depends, by definition, upon a cluster of signs and symptoms, how does the nurse respond if one or two are missing? Nursing diagnosis could lead to an all-or-nothing interpretation in which the diagnosis is not made because one sign is absent or another is not obvious. The patient's problem may therefore be ignored because it does not present in a classical way.

These authors strongly support the views of writers such as Benner, that experienced nurses employ a wide range of skills, including something that may be recognized as intuition, and frequently operate outside the formal rules of deductive logic that fit the nursing process model. The use of more personal and intuitive methods to supplement and build upon the nursing process foundation leads to a much more reflective approach to nursing care. Rew and Barrow point out that this open-minded and creative approach to care can lead to individualized nursing interventions, although the quality audit methods that focus on process and nursing process documentation cannot do justice to quality of such nursing. If more emphasis was placed upon the outcomes of nursing care, or if the quantitative nursing process-based audit tools were rejected, this would be less of a problem and perhaps the 'expert' approach described above would receive the credit it deserves.

Another way of trying to visualize how expert nurses work might be to refer back to the discussion in Chapter 4 concerning Lewin's force field theory of change. It is no coincidence that Lewin was strongly associated with the Gestalt theorists. Figure 10.1 shows a model of a patient's health status. There are forces driving change in the direction of improving health which include family members, therapists and their interventions, doctors and the whole armoury of medical interventions from surgery to medication and, most importantly, the nurse working with the patient's own bodily and psychological resources. But there are forces resisting health change such as patient attitudes, beliefs and other psychological factors, environmental influences and lifestyle factors, social influences, the side-effects of treatment, pathological processes and, of course, family members can be on this side of the line as well. The patient's health status depends upon the balance between these opposing forces and the way they interact.

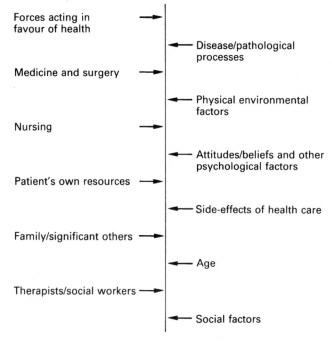

Figure 10.1 *Health and the balance of forces. A patient's health status represents the balance between these two sets of forces.*

The nurse has to intervene in this entire field of forces in order to promote health and recovery. Given the complexity of this situation and the way so many forces connect with others, can we reasonably expect to achieve results by splitting the patient up into individual problems and then working on each problem in a linear fashion? The expert nurse does not do this: s/he sees the whole field of forces and works with the patient to try and move the dividing line towards a position of better health. Military analogies might be inappropriate in a book written about caring, but it is easy to see this model in terms of a battlefield where there are two sets of opposing forces working for and against the patient's health and the individual's current health status is represented by the 'front line' marking the boundary between these opposing forces.

In real battles the front is not a straight line. It is marked by salients where strong positions push into enemy territory but there are weaknesses where ground has been lost. The front is not stagnant; it changes from day to day. The good general seeks to shore up and hold the weak positions on the one hand and exploit his strengths on the other. Attacks probe one part of the front today but switch to another tomorrow if little progress is made. Opportunities are exploited as they present themselves to push at weaknesses while resources are husbanded and not squandered on attacking strongpoints unless absolutely necessary, and only then after maximum preparation. This flexible, changing pattern of activity seems much more akin to what is happening in patient care, as the nurse has an intuitive grasp of the whole field, recalling previous experience, looking for patterns and similarities to previous situations, using common sense and nursing skills to work with the patient towards a successful outcome and, by analogy, a favourable peace.

The example in Figure 10.2 concerns a patient who has been admitted to coronary care with a medical diagnosis of acute myocardial infarction. The original position is shown in Figure 10.2a: this represents the baseline on admission and initial assessment. The various forces at work can be seen to produce a moving front line, reflecting the changing health status of the patient. The expert nurse sees the whole picture and works with the patient and other health professionals such as medical staff and physiotherapists to improve health by maybe holding the line in some sections whilst moving forward in others. Progress made in some sections then allows the nurse to switch attention to other

(a) *Base-line status*

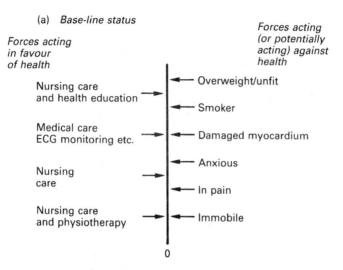

(b) *24 hours after admission*

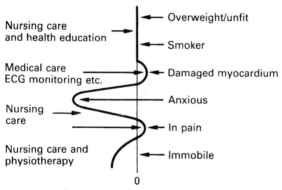

Nursing care has been unable to deal with patient anxiety and ground has been lost. Pain has been relieved and the ECG stabilized, representing progress, although the patient remains on bed rest. There has been no change in weight or smoking habits in the immediate short term as health education has not commenced.

Figure 10.2 *Example of how a patient's health status changes in response to a range of forces. Patient has been admitted with an acute myocardial infarction. The bold line represents health status*

(c) *5 days after admission*

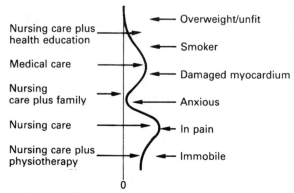

Progress is being made along the front but at different rates in different places.
From a quality point of view. → = process; ⟩ = outcomes.

(d) *3 months after admission*

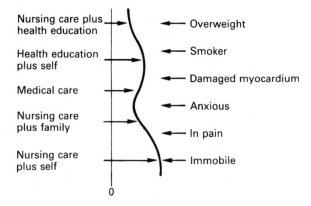

A major move towards increased health status has occurred as a result of forces acting in favour of health, pushing back the forces resisting this movement. Of course, new forces may come into play to help or hinder the move towards improved health status.

Figure 10.2 *(continued)*

areas slightly later. The result is a gradual advance, though by no means in a regular and smooth fashion, until at discharge the patient's health has been moved to a much more favourable position than on admission. It is possible to summarize a patient's progress in this fashion and readers are invited to try, using some patients they have nursed recently.

To stay with the military metaphor, the rigid implementation of the nursing process is reminiscent of Haigh's generals in World War I, who believed that an army can just survey the ground, lay its plans, then advance steadily, on all fronts simultaneously and in one direction, by a logical process of attrition all the way to Berlin (Fig. 10.3). Devotees of Rowan Atkinson's Captain Blackadder character will be familiar with the cunning plans of Private Baldrick: they had as much chance of success as those of the generals. The graves of Flanders bear silent testimony to this failure of imagination.

The analogy described above offers a view of experienced nursing which is much more complex than the step-by-step plodding of the nursing process. The patient is seen as being at the centre of this complex interplay of opposing forces, health status is the front line and the nurse acts as the general, working with the patient to roll back ill health in a complex and sensitive way. Total victory is rarely possible in war and so it is in the struggle for health. However, a relative victory which the patient recognizes as progress can be just as important, and even more important perhaps because it is achievable. That is the strength of nursing – acknowledging that total victory (i.e. cure) is rarely possible. Instead, nurses work with the patient to secure a favourable and achievable peace.

Nurses are therefore being oppressed by the constraints of the nursing process, unable to express themselves freely and develop new ways of approaching care that are the very essence of nursing. It is the traditional scientific world view which is articulated specifically by the medical profession that devalues care. Smith (1991) draws attention to the work of various feminist writers who have argued that caring is devalued as a result of being seen as women's work and therefore a low status rather than the higher-status, male-dominated technical work such as medicine. The skills of caring, including the emotional labour of not showing feelings on the outside in order to present a calm, reassuring exterior, are therefore not recognized by those in power.

Benner and Wrubel (1989) offer the powerful definition of care as understanding the lived experience of illness. The nurse in their view 'presences' him or herself with patients in such a way as to try and share their humanity. This view challenges the detached, scientific methodology of the nursing process in its conventional format as a valid way of planning care for expert nurses. Society, as it has become more competitive and individualistic, has devalued caring and in the process nursing, according to these authors. They point to the general view that in some strange way knowledge is aloof from situations, therefore experts cannot get involved and those who are involved cannot be experts. This again devalues nurses who are always involved and challenges the detached, objective view of the nursing process referred to earlier.

Rew and Barrow (1989) go further and consider that the close association of nursing diagnosis and standard-setting with the nursing process also leads to these two areas of nursing activity being subject to the same criticism.

The nursing process is firmly rooted in conventional science but this too has recently been forced to deal with a major challenge to its conventional wisdom, emanating from the proponents of chaos theory. This was introduced in Chapter 4 and one of the characteristics of this new way of thinking about science is known as sensitive dependence upon initial conditions (Gleick, 1987). This notion suggests that if a system exists in such a way that consequences depend very much upon the initial set of conditions, then minor fluctuations in the early stages of the system can be magnified through time and space to produce immense and unpredictable results. The nursing process suffers from this problem. Because it is laid out as a linear process in which every stage depends upon the one before, sensitive dependence upon initial conditions is built into the system. The implication is that if the nurse makes a minor error in the initial patient assessment, the consequences of that error may be multiplied through the process (see Figure 10.4).

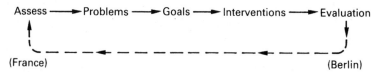

Figure 10.3   *The nursing process represented diagrammatically as a linear process*

Consider the elderly patient who is noted by the nurse to be a little agitated and confused. The problem identification and goal-setting that follow may lead to a decision to request the doctor to write up a minor tranquillizer. This is given, with the result that the patient becomes more confused and disoriented, leading to more frequent administration, resulting in a patient who is awake and disturbed all night and asleep all day. Independence has vanished, self-care is minimal, the patient refuses to drink and becomes dehydrated, constipation is followed by faecal incontinence associated with spurious diarrhoea, the family are distressed, confusion increases, wandering one night the patient falls and fractures the upper femur, surgery follows – leading to a totally dependent patient requiring intensive nursing care who has lost all dignity and contact with reality.

This chapter of disasters is all too familiar, yet in the first place if the nurse had got the assessment right and realized that the patient was perhaps disoriented by the process of hospitalization or had noted signs indicating the beginnings of a chest infection leading to cerebral hypoxia and consequently some mild degree of confusion, interventions would have been very different and would have dealt successfully with the whole patient and the causes of the health problems displayed. Instead, a focus on one aspect of behaviour only and a lack of investigation and critical reflection set in motion a whole chain of disasters as the tranquillizer makes the patient drowsy, and thus increases disorientation. Alternatively, it could act to decrease chest expansion (making the chest infection worse) and air intake (making cerebral hypoxia worse), thereby increasing confusion.

This linear way of thinking – if this, then that – is characteristic of the scientific method but can have disastrous results, because one slight error can be multiplied throughout the system with totally unpredictable results. If the reader pauses to reflect for a few seconds, we feel it is likely you will recall patients where everything seemed to go wrong. One thing led to another. We suggest that this linear way of thinking might be responsible rather than just bad luck. It is of course the way medicine works as well, so that the medical and nursing teams are both operating with the same method and are prone to the same potential error. Paradoxically, many patients may have been saved from this sort of nursing medical-induced chapter of disasters because the nurse actually did not operate in this mechanistic way, despite what was written in the care plan. A nursing Gestalt – an ability to grasp the whole situation and recognize what was necessary rather than a

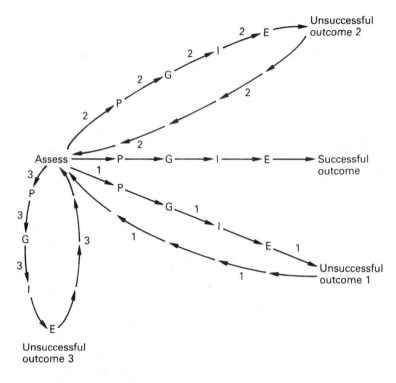

P = problems; G = goals; I = interventions; = E = evaluation.

Once the process has got off on the wrong direction it will continue going in the wrong direction and possibly move further and further away the desired successful outcome in an unpredictable way, as routes 1, 2 and 3 show. The process has to go all the way to an unsuccessful outcome before returning to the beginning and starting all over again.

Figure 10.4   *How it can go wrong if the process starts in the wrong direction*

narrow reductionist, linear approach, as exemplified by the nursing process – may permit many nurses to avoid this trap, whilst presenting them with the difficulty of having to appear to conform to the nursing process model.

Conclusions

These last two chapters have discussed at length the problems associated with care-planning. Nursing diagnoses have been rejected whilst nursing models are acknowledged as having liberating possibilities, as well as the unfortunate potential to be used as a means of coercing nursing into a narrow perspective of care.

The nursing process approach developed out of education where it was found to be a useful method of teaching students and does assist newly qualified nurses in their first year or so of practice. However, experience has shown that it is not appropriate for experienced nurses as it simply does not fit the way they tend to work. It devalues clinical expertise and, in seeking to mimic medicine, only propagates nursing's subordination. When presented as the sole method of planning care it excludes large areas of the health-care agenda from nursing's attention and in that sense can also be used as a means of controlling what nurses think and do. There is little evidence that nurses use it in any real way to involve patients in their own care.

The liberation of nursing therefore requires recognition that the nursing process is ultimately unhelpful for many experienced nurses. Before throwing the kardex in the bin, however, awkward facts remain. Care given must be organized; it must be documented for future reference and if the patient-centred, primary nursing philosophy is to be followed, documentation which clearly links care prescribed with the nurse responsible must exist.

The long-winded, hand-written approach to care-planning should be dropped on the grounds that it frequently bears little resemblance to care given, it consumes inordinate amounts of nursing time and it is based upon a system that does not match the way expert nurses operate. Nurses should be freed to develop their own systems of recording care, one of which might be the use of pre-written units of care. These can be computer-stored, and swiftly assembled in the light of detailed assessment to make a plan outlining the principles of care required. Such units of care should be prepared in conjunction with other professional health-care staff such as physiotherapists and occupational therapists to ensure that a coordinated approach is taken to care. This gives junior staff a framework to work with. It also gives the senior nurse responsible for care the time to individualize this framework to the patient's needs.

The plan of care therefore is not a detailed, hand-written statement of the obvious; rather it is about principles of care and focuses on outcomes. This gives the expert nurse the freedom to care for the patient according to his/her Gestalt view of the whole patient and his or her changing daily health status. The expert nurse does what is necessary. Progress notes need only reflect what is considered important; the nurse is not forced to record routine and spurious information in a hundred and one boxes and columns. A blank sheet of paper for progress reports might be the best documentation.

A standard-setting approach to quality assurance will do much to ensure that the process of care achieves acceptable standards rather than a laboriously written care plan which is ignored most of the time. Focus on outcomes of care acknowledges the nurses's accountability for care delivered. The details of how the nurse and patient completed the journey from admission to discharge become relatively less important: what matters is the patient's health status on discharge either from hospital or from care altogether. Where the journey ends becomes more important and how the patient got there relatively less so, although research that investigates which interventions might be more effective than others still has to be recognized as important.

The obsession with recording every minute detail of care reflects the traditional nursing administrator's lack of trust of clinical staff. The medicolegal importance of progress notes cannot be denied; however, they are frequently of such poor quality that there would appear to be little to lose and much to gain by encouraging clinical nurses to start again, looking at how they wish to plan and record care on an individualized basis. Such an initiative will empower both nurses and patients, especially if care is truly patient-centred and involves the consumer. The ritual of the nursing process has

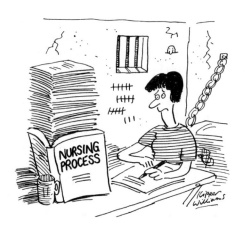

become a prison for nursing – it is time we organized an escape committee and started digging some tunnels.

References

Benner P (1984) *From Novice to Expert*. Menlo Park, Addison Wesley.

Benner P, Wrubel J (1989) *The Primary of Caring*. Menlo Park, Addison Wesley.

Benner P, Tanner C (1987) Clinical judgement: how expert nurses use intuition. *American Journal of Nursing* 87: 23–31.

Freire P (1985) *The Politics of Education, Culture, Power and Liberation* (translated by Macedo C). New York, Macmillan.

Gleick J (1987) *Chaos*. New York, Cardinal.

Habermas J (1976) *Communication and the Evolution of Society* (translated by McCarthy T). Boston, Beacon Press.

Hiraki A (1992) Tradition, rationality and power in introductory nursing textbooks: a critical hermeneutics study. *Advances in Nursing Science* 14: 1–12.

Hurst K, Dean A, Trickey S (1991) The recognition and non-recognition of problem solving stages in nursing practice. *Journal of Advanced Nursing* 16: 1444–1455.

Pyles S, Stern P (1983) Discovery of nursing Gestalt in critical care nursing. *Image: The Journal of Nursing Scholarship* 15: 51–57.

Rew L (1988) Intuition in decision making. *Image: The Journal of Nursing Scholarship* 20: 150–154.

Rew L, Barrow M (1989) Nurses' intuition. *AORN Journal* 50: 353–358.

Schraeder B, Fischer D (1987) Using intuitive nursing in the neo-natal intensive care nursery. *Holistic Nursing Practice* 1: 45–51.

Schon D (1983) *The Reflective Practitioner*. New York, Basic Books.

Smith P (1991) The nursing process: raising the profile of emotional care in nurse training. *Journal of Advanced Nursing* 16: 74–81.

11 *A case study of nursing empowerment*

Introduction

This penultimate chapter looks at what can happen when a group of ordinary nursing staff in a provincial hospital, working in a care of the elderly unit, get together and decide to change things. It demonstrates the latent power that is so often untapped within nursing which can bring about significant changes in care, providing that staff feel confident enough to try and be different. It does not need Nursing Development Unit status, nor does it require any high-powered academic involvement or the presence of any messianic figurehead. However, it does need clinical experience and a willingness to hold that experience up for critical reflection. Imagination and a little daring also help.

The group of nurses in this study worked on a care of the elderly unit and were endeavouring to provide individualized care but felt that none of the common nursing models currently on offer met their needs, so they wondered if they could develop their own model of care. That was the starting point for this work. Such a model could provide a framework for care, while its evolution in the light of practical experience would facilitate the essential linkage of theory and practice.

This chapter describes the development of an approach to care by a group of clinical nurses who believed there was a need for a model which was derived from the experiences of 'hands-on' clinical nurses and which was particularly suited to the needs of elderly people. Such an approach to care would be required to uphold the key values of nurses working with elderly people, in addition to the more general nursing values. An alternative approach, consisting of taking pieces from different models and fitting them together, was rejected initially as this felt artificial and messy. It was like trying to put together a complete outfit by searching through several different people's wardrobes and trying to match bits and pieces together.

The philosophy of care that is presented in this chapter is built upon the values of nurses who work with elderly people in both acute and rehabilitation areas. These values are based upon the premise that the individual wishes to live a normal and independent life within society and the need therefore to recognize this requirement at all times when the person is hospitalized. This exercise made the nurses who developed this model examine their own values and beliefs. Such an exercise is essential in any attempt to build a consensus which leads to an agreed philosophy of care.

The staff found that, in collecting together and discussing their values and beliefs, each member had his or her own independent approach to nursing practice based upon his or her own value system. This demonstrates the importance of this crucial first step of sharing views and opinions about care, for only in this way can agreement be reached around a common philosophy. Failure to do so leads to a wide range of sometimes conflicting and often confusing approaches which mitigates against teamwork and may cause distress to patients and families alike. Such a sharing, consensus-building approach is the first step towards empowerment.

The staff quickly realized that the experience of working together to design and test out their own model of care could change attitudes and beliefs whilst leading to further development of professional practice in all concerned. A key point was the need for the systematic construction of the model in such a way that at all times the group were striving to make clear the nurse's role in care delivery. This crucial point is the subject of much intense debate at present and nurses must never lose sight of their unique professional position.

Recognizing the need for change

Many years ago, the members of this group were, with the help of a half study day, required to implement the nursing processes. All qualified staff had a training session which concentrated on the new documentation. Questions were met with confusing answers, which suggested that there was at that stage a lack of understanding amongst those delivering the session concerning just what the nursing process involved. Students appeared to have received a rather sketchy introduction to 'the process' as some students denied all knowledge of it at the time whilst others did manage to demonstrate some understanding of the basic notions involved. The situation will be familiar to many readers – staff trying to care for patients in a climate of change but with inadequate information about and understanding of whatever the changes are.

Since those early days, staff in the elderly care unit have worked hard, struggling to document individual client needs amongst familiar mutterings to the effect: 'But this is nothing new, we have always given individualized care'.

For some this was indeed true; skilled, perceptive and sensitive nurses did give a substantial amount of individualized care within the constraints of service provision. It was apparent, though, that continuity in care was not being achieved, however this care was documented. The situation was exacerbated by the differing and idiosyncratic interpretations that various nurses placed upon the nursing process, which resulted in a variety of styles of care plan documentation, few of which stated specific objectives in achievable steps. This led to confusion amongst staff, fragmentation of care and loss of motivation and commitment.

As a forward-looking department, methods of clinical practice and management were being continually evaluated and updated, with the result that when discussions about nursing models began in the UK, the staff wondered if models could assist with the nursing process difficulties. A very searching visit from the English National Board convinced the department that they could no longer just complacently accept the 'problems with the process' – something had to be done. After all, the department had well-motivated and keen staff who read extensively and who discussed current issues in nursing, including the emerging nursing models literature. Was this the answer?

At the time some of the wards were using a guide based around common daily living activities to facilitate care plan completion. The following familiar headings made up the guide:

- Transfers.
- Mobility.
- Washing.
- Dressing.
- Toileting.
- Clothing management during toileting.
- Eating.
- Drinking.

- Pressure areas.
- Communication.
- Mental state.

Although very physically biased, the staff had the beginnings of an approach to care in so far as there was a framework which placed some structure upon practice. There was of course no philosophy of care as yet, just a list of headings, but it was a beginning.

As staff began to explore the skills and values of nursing at this time in informal discussions, it became apparent that the whole 24 hours of the patient's day needed to be considered in terms of patterns of care. What did nurses do and when? How did they relate to the multidisciplinary team? What resources were used and to what ends? Questions such as these led to the identification of ritualistic and rigid practice. Uppermost in the minds of those staff engaged in this reflective and critical process was the realization that individualized care had been a struggle because they had never before truly examined their role as nurses, nor had they considered whether they shared a common philosophy of care. Staff realized that they had no coherent framework or agreed philosophy to guide practice; it was like trying to drive from Lands End to John O'Groats with no idea of the route.

This demonstrates how sharing views and experiences in an open and equal framework within which critical reflection upon practice is encouraged can lead to real progress, change and both personal and professional growth. Staff now began exploring models as potentially helpful and useful ways of improving care if they could rectify some of the problems that had been identified. They were not seeing them as yet another 'North American flavour-of-the-month fad' being imposed by management.

Discussion led to the realization that there were elements in several different models which were very attractive, with Orem's self-care model seeming to have the most relevance. In the subsequent development work it can be seen that Orem's work had the biggest single influence on the team. The preference, however, was to try and develop an approach to care unique to the unit in question, as this would give all the staff a sense of ownership and achievement, in addition to being customized to meet the needs of patients on the unit. Staff were aware that growing their own model was a huge undertaking in terms of time and effort but were excited at the challenge and aware that this represented a tremendous learning opportunity for all.

The approach taken consisted of attempting to build a model out of clinical experience rather than theoretical abstractions. This model would be one firmly rooted in practice rather than relying upon academically rigorous knowledge. This has much in common with the methods discussed in Chapter 3.

The first attempts at brainstorming values and beliefs in order to arrive at a common philosophy were stimulating but failed to achieve an early agreement. However, there was a consensus around Virginia Henderson's well-known philosophy:

The unique function of the nurse is to assist the individual, sick or well, in the performance of those activities contributing to health or its recovery (or to a peaceful death) that he would peform unaided if he had the necessary strength, will or knowledge and to do this in such a way as to help him gain independence as rapidly as possible (Henderson, 1966).

With agreement reached upon this as a first stage in developing a philosophy, the next step was to arrive at a consensus view of what was understood by a model. The following definition emerged: 'a model is a collection of ideas about people's needs and how best to fulfil them'. In addition a model could act as an overall plan which would guide nurses' thinking. The function of the model would be to enable the nurse, in partnership with the patient and family, to carry out a thorough assessment of health needs and produce a meaningful plan of care. This was the view that the staff worked with throughout and it is different from some of the academic definitions that may be found in other texts. It is the definition used in this chapter and what mattered was that the staff had a definition that they could agree on rather than an imposed textbook definition which may not command universal support. All things in life are relative, including the meaning of a nursing model.

Action to develop the model

At this stage the staff had achieved a consensus upon the following:

- An understanding of what models of nursing are.
- Models could facilitate individualized patient care.
- The need to develop a model unique to the unit.

- A first step in developing a philosophy of care would be Virginia Henderson's definition of nursing.

The starting point for developing the model was a consideration of human needs within society. This had to be health- rather than ill-health-oriented, which was a problem for some members of staff, who were still strongly influenced by the medical model of illness. The whole group were involved in brainstorming sessions that consumed large quantities of flipchart paper and pens in a stimulating and creative exercise. Great care was taken to ensure a secure and safe environment for this work.

Six main patient needs emerged from this work:

1. Psychological.
2. Social.
3. Economic.
4. Physical
5. Environmental.
6. Spiritual.

To maintain the momentum and expedite the work on these headings the group divided into six subgroups, each taking a topic to explore before the next meeting. Much frantic activity ensued during the following week, with many members of staff contributing their thoughts to the subgroups' deliberations.

When the subgroups reconvened, the discussion was led by a staff nurse in each case. All the presentations were constructively questioned and debated until a consensus emerged about the principal needs identified by each subgroup. At this stage it was apparent that there was substantial overlap between the topics. The team were also aware of the criticism that, whilst striving to achieve a holistic view of nursing care, the work was fragmenting the patient into different areas.

In order to resolve the problems of overlap and fragmentation, the next step was to convene a meeting at which the flipcharts were spread on the floor so that all participants could see at once what the other subgroups had achieved. This was followed by an examination of the nature of the nurse–patient relationship in order to identify specific needs which flowed from this interaction. These could then be compared with the list of general needs outlined above. The team identified the following patient needs:

- Individuality.
- Freedom of choice.
- Security and safety.
- Comfort.
- Dignity.
- Self-esteem.
- Uniqueness.
- Maintenance of health.
- Continuity of care.

The less-experienced members of the group began to realize the full importance of individualized care as they tried to reconcile these two sets of needs. Consideration of the second list led to the realization that there were three key concepts that the nurse had to recognize before making any significant interventions in these areas of need. These were:

1. Observation.
2. Communication.
3. Orientation.

Observation

The act of observation involves the collection and recording of information. Criticism has been levelled against the nursing process because of the substantial amount of time required for this activity. The team therefore believed in the importance of recording only relevant, concise, understandable and usable information concerning the patient's needs.

Communication

It became apparent that the concept of communication was crucial as, without it, information concerning the patient's needs could neither be transmitted nor received. Communication (both verbal and non-verbal) was also noted to involve all the senses.

Orientation

Unless patients were familiar with their environment, they could not be expected to feel at ease and derive maximum therapeutic benefit from their hospital stay. This concept should be extended to ensure that the patient is oriented in time and, most importantly, to person. Orientation ensures that the patient feels secure in an environment that could otherwise be very alien and intimidating. Security thus facilitates meeting patient needs.

Having identified these three key concepts that would underpin their approach to care, the team then went on to develop four key statements of belief about the care of elderly people. These statements may be summarized as a belief in:

- Acceptance of the person as an individual and recognition of his/her needs.
- The individual's freedom of choice within the confines of a therapeutic environment.
- The promotion of health, self-esteem and well-being of the individual.
- A joint nurse–patient approach to the identification and solution of problems.

It was now possible to identify a philosophy that would underpin the evolving model of care and which encompassed these beliefs. This philosophy may be summarized as follows:

The individual is a unique being who responds to environmental stimuli in such a way as to meet his/her needs. These needs are not reduced by illness. The nurse/carer must accept the individuality of the patient and, through partnership, assist the individual in meeting his/her requirements, thereby promoting health.

As work progressed, the initial lists discussed above changed and altered, becoming absorbed into new concepts which finally grew into a new approach to care on the unit.

Before considering how these concepts subsequently evolved, it is worth noting that this philosophy was a straightforward statement of commonly held beliefs that all the team could support. To criticize it as merely a statement of the obvious is to miss the point. It was an essential step in developing care on the unit as previously, when staff had each followed their own views, the result had been confusing and at times contradictory. Such a statement therefore gets all the staff pulling in the same direction at the same time.

Working from the insight that orientation, communication and observation were three key nursing activities, the next step was to ask what might be seen as key patient activities? The empowering philosophy discussed above would provide the link between the two.

Some lateral thinking and brainstorming from experience suggested two broad headings – dynamics and mechanics. Dynamics represented to these nurses the everyday processes of our intellectual and emotional selves: moods, emotions, feelings and thoughts. They are things which flow and change, sometimes with the unpredictability and turbulence of the eddies and whirlpools seen in the flow of a river. The river can do something else, however; it can work a waterwheel. It was this notion of the everyday work of life that led the group to conceptualize mechanics as meaning movement and effort. Such work needs fuel such as food, fluids and the intake of oxygen, which in their turn produce the waste products of metabolism which have to be disposed of by elimination. Health problems of course affect our abilities to carry out these functions and at this stage the nurses working on the project acknowledged their debt to Dorothea Orem's concept of self-care abilities, which fitted their philosophy and was consistent with the view of nursing for the older person that the team were trying to develop.

Slowly but surely, the broad outlines were emerging of an approach to nursing that met the requirements of the team and which seemed consistent with the needs of their client group. It was apparent, though, that so far the team had not addressed the issues of personal choice for the client and also the safeguarding of privacy, dignity and personal space, or, to summarize, the client's own territory while in hospital. By now the group had almost made a word with the initial letters of these various concepts – CCOMODAT. It was easy to see that if an A was added on the front to represent the first thing that happens to a patient, admission, and an E to the end to represent the hoped-for destination of the patient, the home environment, the nursing team could easily summarize their view of the keys to successful nursing care for the older person by the mnemonic ACCOMODATE.

A Admission – the entry into hospital care which must be handled sensitively and which links to other concepts such as observation and orientation.

C Communication – important at admission and at all stages thereafter if there is to be a true partnership with the patient which addresses individual needs.

C   Choice – something the patient must have at all times as part of the empowering, equal partnership approach to care that characterizes the chosen philosophy.

O   Observation – continual observation of the whole patient is essential. This means much more than vital signs monitoring.

M   Mechanics – the physical work of life, movement, dexterity and the fuels they require: nutrition, fluid and air intake, eliminatory functions.

O   Orientation – to time, place and person. This is a major concern in care of the older person.

D   Dynamics – the emotional, intellectual and spiritual aspects of the patient are conceptualized under this heading.

A   Abilities – independence and self-care ability in terms of personal hygiene, feeding, etc.

T   Territory – personal space and integrity, belongings and memories, the recognition of personal dignity.

E   Environment – particularly outside hospital, the importance of where the patient has come from and where he or she is returning.

The nurses who participated in this work had identified from their own extensive experience of working with elderly people a series of key concepts that were essential to a holistic philosophy of care. This was the beginnings of an approach to care, derived from practice rather than deduced from theory, that reflected the ideals and aims of practitioners. This is not a finished product, a well-honed, intellectually watertight and elegant academic treatise that can be called a theory of nursing. It is not characterized by scientific logic or deductive reasoning and therefore does not conform to the rules of technical rationality (see Chapter 3). What it is, though, is a statement of things that matter in the real world, an approach to nursing that recognizes priorities of care which the ward team all share and which is capable of development into a nursing model based around real human needs and empowerment in the elderly care environment.

A crucial aspect of this development is that it works in practice and keeps on working; it has not fizzled out after a few months once the initial enthusiasm has waned. Evaluation has shown that it meets the needs of patients and staff. Students, interestingly, are typically critical of ACCOMODATE when it is first introduced because it lacks an obvious theoretical base, unlike other models they might encounter. Experience brings about a marked change in attitude as they find it user-friendly and appropriate for the needs of the patients. Perhaps this is an example of cognitive dissonance theory at work?

A key observation about this initiative is that the nurses had empowered each other in carrying out this work whose conclusion was an approach to care that stressed empowering the patient. This linkage is no coincidence.

The staff have since developed care-planning documentation which reflects the above main areas of concern. They are characterized by putting the most important things first, so the first thing a nurse sees when picking up an individual's care plan is information concerning orientation, principal facts concerning admission, such as next of kin, previous hospital admission and the individual's perceptions of the need for hospitalization and key nursing observations, according to the client's needs. Within the plan of care, an enabling philosophy, focusing upon self-care abilities is apparent whilst the assessment of the client moves into the areas of choice, communication, mechanics, dynamics and self-care abilities. These principles, along with respect for the individual as an equal partner, drive the nursing care on the ward from admission to discharge planning.

A great deal of change was involved in the way the unit worked as these ideas were implemented. This change from removing the obvious ritualistic and time-wasting aspects of care through to completely changing the care documentation forms. Crucially, though, there was a change in the way staff thought about and planned care, now placing the patient at the centre of activity. Nurses took responsibility for patients by utilizing the concept of primary nursing. Education of staff concerning the new ideas was greatly facilitated by the fact that the staff felt they owned the ideas, as indeed they did, having assisted in their development. Workshops were arranged on a unit basis for the benefit of trained staff and then, utilizing the cascade concept, they in their turn organized ward-based workshops for nursing assistant staff. Change has occurred in this unit with the active participation of all grades of staff utilizing an educative–normative process. The old system was unfrozen by the recognition of the need for change, which then took place by the process of involving as many people as possible.

The authors of this work would not claim that their work has progressed smoothly and is a model of excellence. However, there has been real change and a great sense of progress in the unit which has been achieved by clinically based nurses using expertise derived first-hand from practice, coupled with the will to succeed in their aim of improving services for older people.

Evaluation of staff attitudes and morale before and after the changes were implemented over a 12-month period and has been very encouraging. Staff in the unit were asked to rate their satisfaction on a scale of 0–10 for a wide range of aspects of their work. Response rates were 70% on the questionnaires for both studies and the mean scores were 4.8 before the implementation of the new approach to care: 6 months after, this had risen to 7.7. Of interest was the observation that the care characteristic that improved most referred to the degree of patient orientation; this went from 3.3 to 7.9, while in the area of choice that was available, ratings here went from a mean of 3.9 to 7.3. The dramatic improvement in staff morale revealed by these figures needs to be monitored on an ongoing basis, however, for there is bound to be a degree of novelty which is exerting a favourable influence on these ratings. Attitudes also showed a marked shift towards a greater recognition of client choice, dignity and privacy, which fed through into a more positive feeling about the value of individualized care-planning.

This account demonstrates that clinical staff can change practice providing they work in a mutually supportive and empowering way that involves honest and critical reflection upon practice. In the previous chapter we suggested that the intelligent use of computer-generated care plans may be of benefit in improving individualized care. The nurses in this study have achieved a major improvement without such computer resources. It must be acknowledged that unthinking and ritualistic following of computerized care plans will not improve individualized care.

If staff feel secure in a group, they will dare to be different and throw up unconventional ways of thinking and conceptualizing patient care, as the nurses did in this account. A new approach to care can be developed out of practice rather than textbooks and because staff feel they are stakeholders in this innovation, they are likely to be more willing to accept any associated changes. Perhaps this is a case where the process of change is at least as informative as the outcome.

The work described here has not been the subject of a major formal evaluation, but if readers wish to know more they may contact Helen Peace, Senior Nurse, Elderly Services Directorate, Ipswich General Hospital, Ipswich, Suffolk. She will be happy to supply a detailed resource pack with details of documentation. Please enclose an A4-size stamped addressed envelope and a cheque for £10, payable to the Elderly Services Directorate, to cover the expense of the pack.

Reference

Henderson V (1966) *The Nature of Nursing*. London, Collier-Macmillan.

12 *Reflections*

Nursing today faces its biggest challenge since Nightingale's revolution a century ago. Ironically, this crisis stems at least in part from nursing's own success in the 1970s and 1980s at developing its professional independence and challenging conventional power structures in health care. From the mid 1980s onwards nursing has been under attack from powerful political and managerial authorities driven by an unholy alliance of ideology and financial constraints, whilst also contending with the familiar doctor–nurse power struggle. When more general social forces are added to this mixture, such as sex role stereotyping which tends to discriminate against women, the result is a profession under attack.

Reading the weekly nursing press can be a very depressing affair as the news is of redundancies amongst nurses and ward closures while the numbers of administrative and clerical staff increase as the new NHS trusts stagger from one financial crisis to another. It is not surprising to read reports of falling morale and despondency amongst nurses. Through all of this runs the constant theme of change which seems to be occurring at an ever-accelerating pace and with little regard to the views of the professional staff who work in the service. Teachers are another group who are undergoing a similar experience.

This turbulent and rapidly changing scene leads us as authors to want to hold on to this manuscript for a little longer to see how some latest new development unfolds and then another and then another. The book would never be published, of course, if we did that so the time has come to draw a line under what we have said, conscious for example that the UKCC document on *Post-Registration Education and Practice* will have been out for consultation and hopefully agreement on the way forward will have been reached by the time this book is in the shops. The initial response of the profession to the document was, however, very critical and it is clear that the UKCC needs to reconsider its plans seriously.

We have advocated the concept of the reflective practitioner in this text so it is appropriate for us to finish by reflecting back on what we have written. This book began with the authors' concern that potentially exciting and beneficial nursing developments might become devalued and ritualized whilst other new ideas were being enthusiastically and uncritically embraced without being subject to critical scrutiny. In warning of false messiahs who simplistically appear to have all the answers, we make no such claims ourselves. This text urges nurses to accept nothing without question and therefore readily invites debate and questions of itself.

The importance of educating nurses to be critical thinkers is crucial, yet there is a danger that post-registration education may become obsessed with technical competencies and become more National Vocational Qualification than intellectually driven. Statements from the UKCC that see post-registration education producing nurse *specialists* are therefore regrettable as this narrows the focus and leads predominantly to competency-based education. The importance of technical skills is not denied, but there must be more to post-registration nursing education than reinventing the old task-focused style of nurse training that Project 2000 is trying to get away from. This point is particularly salient in view of the fact that most registered nurses had precisely such a task-focused, uncritical basic training. Unless educators devise post-registration programmes designed to lead nurses towards developing as critical thinkers, rituals will continue to flourish and new ideas will be uncritically accepted.

This critical approach to post-registration education has been called emancipatory teaching by Burrows (1993); she describes this as aiming to empower students by allowing them to develop and articulate their own ideas. Critical thinking involves reflection and reasoning and is encouraged through dialogue between teacher and student. Burrows suggests three strategies which involve clinical judgement seminars, simulations and journal-keeping. The former involves group analysis of critical incidents drawn from the students' own experience in which what actually happened and how things might have been done differently are discussed. Simulation involves giving small groups case studies or situations which require decisions about action and then comparing the different solutions the groups arrive at. Journal-keeping requires the student to spend a few minutes jotting down feelings and ideas about their classwork which helps clarify thinking in the short term and which also makes a valuable resource for future reflection and discussion.

The combination of educational approaches such as these with the necessary more technical, competency-based information is essential if post-registration education is to produce the critical thinkers that were never on traditional nurse-training's agenda. The success of Project 2000 in producing critical thinkers will be impossible to judge for some time but already some writers such as Taylor (1993) are critical of nurse tutors who continue to teach from above in the traditional way and therefore are unlikely to produce nurses who can question and confront conventional nursing wisdom.

Taylor draws upon the writings of Paulo Freire, which have been extensively referred to in this text elsewhere, to argue that nurse tutors should be 'teaching for subversion', i.e. teaching students critically to question the status quo. This style of teaching, she argues, will only come about when students learn through experience rather than being required passively to absorb facts in a classroom bound by hierarchical relationships with tutors. This is what Schon (1987) refers to as a 'practicum', which he defines as 'a setting designed for the task of learning a practice. . . . It stands in an intermediate space between the practice world, the "lay" world of ordinary life, and the esoteric world of the academy'. In nursing, Schon's practicum is not a real building but rather an intellectual environment which surrounds the student in clinical areas with supernumerary status, which allows students to practise skills such as communication or blood pressure measurements upon each other; it is in the library and most importantly within the way that tutors facilitate, rather than direct student exploration of the world of nursing.

The key, according to Taylor, is to promote an assertive self-image in the student as one who can learn continuously in cooperation with others and who is capable of making decisions that can ultimately lead to change. This is the language of empowerment and reflection and the rejection of gender role stereotypes of women, of course. Nursing's future depends upon developing the character-istics discussed in the preceding paragraphs within both pre- and post-registration education.

Nursing education is moving rapidly into the new world of higher education where the critical approaches discussed above are accepted as normal. Nursing is, however, starting from a very low point in this new academic environment. For example, the Flowers

Report (1993) into the structure of the academic year acknowledges the special needs of medicine, initial teacher training and engineering to have non-standard academic years but never mentions nursing once. It appears that the high-powered academics on the panel chaired by Lord Flowers are unaware of nursing's existence in higher education.

Nursing research has been given a very poor rating also within the higher education sector as a result of the University Funding Council's (UFC) assessment that only three out of 29 university sector departments were carrying out research which was of national excellence, while 60% of departments were given the lowest possible ratings (Marsland, 1993). Marsland is critical of prominent nurse researchers who agree with this dismal rating, as they are doing the profession a grave disservice. Higher education is fiercely competitive when resources are at stake and previous ratings in excellence in research are one of the crucial yardsticks used when funds are allocated for future research. The situation may be aptly summed up by a quotation from the Bible:

For everyone who has will be given more and he will have an abundance. Whoever does not have, even what he has will be taken from him (Matthew 25:29).

The UFC seem to work on the principle of giving resources to those who have a good research record at the expense of those who have not. This means that there is a private members' club of institutions and disciplines who are continually given the resources to fund future research and development, whilst those on the outside are denied the chance to show what they can do if they had the resources, as they will never be given the resources. At the moment nursing is on the outside and struggling for access to research funds that could make a major contribution to developing nursing knowledge and hence practice. As Marsland has noted, the way nursing handled the publication of these dismal ratings is selling ourselves short, particularly as the exercise was invalid with regard to nursing anyway.

The development of nursing knowledge from research has therefore been seen as a crucial component of professional evolution. While it is necessary to recognize the importance of academic-based research, as discussed above, it is equally important to remember that a great deal of nursing knowledge derives from reflection upon practice. Schon (1987) strongly argues this case as he sees practitioners developing knowing-in-action through reflection-in-action and that this is equally valid when compared with more formal knowledge generated from research conducted in university departments. Nurses have always talked about common-sense knowledge that will not be found in standard textbooks. It is to this type of knowledge that Schon refers in his attempts to win academic recognition of its value.

Nursing Development Units (NDUs) have attracted a great deal of attention recently, but it would be unfortunate if nurses thought that these were the only alternatives to university departments for the generation of new ideas and nursing knowledge. That way lies the road to élitism. Nurses may develop knowledge about nursing from their nursing practice in any environment. This requires reflection and critical thinking, discussion with colleagues, trying to see alternatives and being willing to experiment. The previous chapter gave an account of how such a project developed in an empowering environment on a care of the elderly unit. The key message is that nursing knowledge can be developed outside of the formal academic research environment or NDUs by nurses working in a wide range of settings.

The jury is still out on the value of NDUs. Critical thinking requires all things to be questioned and there are no taboos. The concept behind NDUs is very positive and empowering but the awkward question of whether NDUs can justify their existence has to be asked. Are some of them in danger of becoming bastions of élitism and egotism that obstruct the empowerment and liberation of the nursing profession by the process of vanguardism which Paulo Freire described in Chapter 3? Critical reflection upon the worth of NDUs and an objective evaluation of care given are essential in the harsh value-for-money climate of today, as well as for the wider philosophical debate surrounding their contribution to nursing knowledge. Much was made of the pioneering role of NDUs in introducing primary nursing, yet its worth still remains undemonstrated – so much so that Leach (1993) can still write that the basic beliefs, tenets and values of primary nursing have not been investigated. Leach argues for a more qualitative approach to get to grips with the meanings of primary nursing for patient and nurse rather than the sterile empirical approach which has so far failed to add significantly to our knowledge on primary nursing.

The attachment to the empirical tradition of 'real science' is proving difficult to dissolve. English (1993) has severely criticized Benner's notions about nursing intuition, accusing her of side-stepping the challenge of objective verification by her claim that intuition is part of the art of nursing rather than a scientific component. That is a little like criticizing somebody who says they cannot measure the weight of an object with a tape measure.

English does give a very plausible account of how expert nurses' apparently intuitive recognition of something being wrong with patients may be understood in cognitive processing terms rather than intuition. He argues that nurses become expert at building up a series of scripts which chart patient progress. They are an account of the usual pattern of progress that would be expected, which permits nurses to recognize instantly when something is not quite right, such as a patient's recovery from surgery or a myocardial infarction. Sometimes we are only aware that there is a clock in a room when it stops ticking as we have become so used to it being there. It is part of our 'script' for being in that room that there is a ticking noise, therefore we do not notice it when it is present: only its absence draws it to our attention as there is now a deviation from the script.

This analogy may well explain a great deal of Benner's apparent nursing intuition, but can it explain all the examples given in her and others' work? English falls into the familiar trap of wanting to force nursing into the constraints of traditional science by his assertion that nursing must be based upon scientific knowledge only and that all procedures must be founded upon empirical research. Whilst not wishing to underestimate the importance of scientific knowledge in nursing, a preoccupation with this approach forecloses consideration of other potentially beneficial approaches to care.

In this book we have attempted to urge nurses to reclaim nursing and liberate the profession from those who would hold us in thrall. In the process we think it is possible to change things and challenge conventional wisdom. Some may have read so far and be thinking that this would be well and fine in an ideal world but in the real world of the cash-starved NHS of today such innovation is all pie in the sky. This need not be so, however, as a North American, and therefore market-driven, analysis of health care by MacDonald (1993) reveals.

MacDonald argues that in a competitive market, innovation must have a benefit to an organization that outweighs cost. Three tests may therefore be applied to see if an innovation gives an organization a competitive advantage. These tests should therefore be applied to any nursing innovation and be used by nurses in constructing a case for change within the current market-driven NHS.

First, does the proposed change add to the economic well-being of the organization? In proposing change, therefore, nurses must address the following sort of issues. Does the innovation increase productivity or staff morale? Can it reduce wastage? If the status of the unit can be improved, this may attract increased resources which could range from increased community support through to winning larger contracts from purchasers of health care. Other sources of income generation might include sales of educational resources.

Cost containment can obviously improve the financial well-being of any organization and the most costly single item is nursing time. Cost containment need not imply reducing the quality of service but rather the opposite. Innovations which make better use of nursing time, such as cutting out the costly and largely ineffective writing of care plans and the introduction of some of the ideas outlined in Chapter 10 are therefore to be encouraged. Targeting high-risk patients for intensive nursing interventions to prevent specific potential problems such as pressure sores is another example of cost containment which is also beneficial to the patient. It is worth noting that administrators and directors of nursing at an American hospital currently stand charged with the manslaughter of two patients who died from 'rotting bedsores and total body infection' (Headlines – American Journal of Nursing, 1993).

The second test that may be applied is whether change gives the organization an element that is unique or rare in the relevant field of practice. To this may be added the concept of whether the community perceives the new idea as something that it wants. Nurses who are trying to persuade management to support innovation therefore need to demonstrate that their idea gives the unit or trust something new or something that the community in the area want and might therefore be expected to support.

The final criterion that MacDonald suggests is whether the innovation places the organization in a leadership position which enhances its position and status and hence attracts resources. The case for persuading management to support change in the competitive environment of the current NHS may be greatly enhanced by using these three themes to help construct the argument.

There is an apparent contradiction in that for most of this book we have talked of empowerment, collaboration and sharing, yet this final chapter ends with talk of competition. There is a need to recognize, however, that this is the real world and sometimes nurses need to utilize the arguments of managers to win the case for nursing with managers. As never before, nursing has to justify every penny that is spent. Therefore the introduction of these approaches to innovation from the North American health system is pertinent to this book. They do not mean however that nurses have to be competitive with each other within any organization.

In the North American system a major expansion in the numbers of nurse practitioners employed in acute hospital settings has been reported (Mallinson, 1993). This is interpreted as being because nurses are showing that within this role they provide high-quality care at an economical price that is allowing hospitals to adjust to a reduced availability of junior medical staff. The NHS faces a similar dilemma as long overdue attempts are made to rationalize junior doctors' hours. There is a great opportunity for UK nurses to develop their clinical practice and, as their US counterparts have done, win the argument for change using the language that managers understand – value for money which also enhances the quality of patient care. It is to be hoped that the statutory bodies in the UK do not hinder this kind of development by failing to understand the liberating concept of the nurse practitioner. We do not need the sort of hierarchy suggested by talk of specialist, enhanced and advanced nurse/midwives.

Liberation first requires recognition of oppression and nursing must awaken to this basic fact of life. Feeling sorry for ourselves and adopting a helpless 'There's nothing that can be done' approach is not the answer, nor is jumping on every bandwagon that passes by in the nursing press. Unquestioning acceptance of new ideas leaves the nurse in equally as dangerous a position as the alternative strategy of imitating an ostrich and refusing to listen to new ideas at all. Either way the end-product is ritualistic care which is carried out because somebody says so and which has no foundation of knowledge or research. If readers put this book down valuing their own profession and worth, with a determination to reclaim nursing for clinical nurses, and with a healthy and critical scepticism for bright new ideas, we will feel happy. However we urge the reader to measure this book by its own yardstick: we are no messiahs or gurus and we do not have simple answers to all the problems of nursing.

The only certainty we are sure of is that nothing is certain – life is too complicated for that.

As a final thought which we suggest might start the reader seriously thinking about rituals both new and old, we would recommend the very successful idea described by Brown (1993) of holding a 'nursing sacred cow contest'. The title is a little unfortunate as it may cause offence to Hindus, and Brown apologized for this in her report, but the idea showed that reflection upon practice can also be fun.

Brown and her colleagues organized a competition which involved all nurses in their hospital entering what they saw as nursing's biggest rituals under three headings – the most time-wasting, the silliest and the oldest rituals. After shortlists were drawn up, the entire staff of the hospital were asked to vote to declare the winners, who received nursing sacred cow mugs as prizes. The winning entries were the policy of stripping *all* beds and changing the linen daily (most time-wasting), removing pyjama bottoms for *all* surgical procedures and investigations (the silliest) and running errands for doctors (the oldest). The result of this exercise was to make staff stop and look at what they were doing and ask why they were doing it and also to set the research agenda for the hospital's newly formed nursing research committee. Perhaps it is time there were a few similar competitions in the UK?

The final words in this book belong not to either of us or to any nurse at all, but rather to the Scottish singer and songwriter Dick Gaughan. He was talking about Scottish mythology and the current political situation with regard to Scottish nationalism when he observed that: 'If you are going to sit and wait for a messiah then you had better get a soft cushion because you are in for a long hard wait!' Bonny Prince Charlie in the end achieved nothing for Scotland except to leave many Scots even more oppressed then before. The alternative to sitting on a soft cushion is standing up together for what we believe in as nurses!

References

Brown G (1993) The sacred cow contest. *Canadian Nurse* **89**: 31–33.
Burrows M (1993) Strategies for staff development. *Canadian Nurse* **89**: 32–34.
English I (1993) Intuition as a function of the expert nurse: a critique of Benner's novice to expert model. *Journal of Advanced Nursing* **18**: 387–393.

Flowers Lord (1993) *Review of the Academic Year; Interim Report for Consultation.* Committee of Enquiry, HEFCE.

Headlines (1993) *American Journal of Nursing* March 9.

Leach M (1993) Primary nursing: autonomy or autocracy? *Journal of Advanced Nursing* **18**: 394–400.

MacDonald M (1993) Quality innovation and cost containment. *Canadian Nurse* **89**: 15–17.

Mallinson M (1993) Nurses as house staff. *American Journal of Nursing* March 7.

Marsland D (1993) Research and destroy. *Nursing Standard* **7**: 32, 45.

Schon D (1987) *Educating the Reflective Practitioner.* San Francisco, Jossey-Bass.

Taylor J (1993) Education can never be neutral: teaching for subversion. *Nursing Education Today* **13**: 69–72.

Index

Accountability, 47
  primary nursing and, 131, 136
  standards and, 112
Action research, 74, 78
Adhocracy, 68
Assertion, 243
  classes, 38
  uniforms and, 13
Assertiveness:
  concept of, 39
  training in, 13
Attitudes, 23
  as knowledge, 60
  changing, 20, 69, 71, 72, 76, 143
  cognitive dissonance theory and,
    20
  culture and, 61
  in nursing, 18
  psychology of, 20
  reasons for, 19
  stress and, 19
  values and, 19
Austen, Jane, 95
Australia, 30
Authoritarian behaviour:
  of ward sisters, 43
Authority:
  acceptance of, 9, 60

Beliefs, 23
  as knowledge, 60
  cognitive dissonance theory and,
    20
  culture and, 61
  in nursing, 18
  psychology of, 20

Budgets:
  nurse's knowledge of, 47

Care and caring:
  acceptable level of, 101
  as changing process, 63
  beliefs and attitudes and, 19
  'chunking' approach to, 69
  creative approach to, 216
  decision-making in, 48
  definition, of, 120, 122
  devaluation of, 85, 222
  equation with task completion,
    36
  for individual patient, 117
  holistic philosophy of, 237
  in male dominated society, 13
  individualized, 183, 184, 193, 199,
    200, 210, 228, 230, 234
    nursing process and, 190
  involvement of patient in, 142
  key concepts, 234
  keys to, 236
  model-guided, 206
  new approach to, 239
  nursing assistants and, 9
  objective evaluation of, 245
  organizing, 182
  outcome and goal of, 51
  partnership in, 134
  patient involvement in, 138
  patient-centred, 45, 121, see also
    Care and caring,
    individualized
  planning, 69, see also Care plans
  primary nursing and, 144

Care and caring (*continued*)
  principles of, 194
    care plans and, 195
  problem-solving approach to, 213
  quality of, *see under* Quality of
    care etc.
  reflective approach to, 216
  staffing requirements, 100, 101
  stress-coping behaviour and, 17
  subordination of, 47
  taken over by social services, 79
  task-centred, 45, 182, 183
  transforming nature of, 120, 121
  units-of-care approach, 197
  value of, 5, 33
Care plans, 181, 225
  alternative approaches to, 192
  becoming ritual, 188
  computers in, 196, 197, 198, 199
  core, 194, 195
  documentation, 238
  handwritten, 195
  language of, 192, 204
  living activities in, 230
  medical terminology in, 192
  need for, 187
  nurses' opinion of, 186
  nursing diagnosis and, 200
  quality of care and, 197
  standardized, 194
  standard-setting and, 195, 198
  unit approach, 197
Change, 42
  approaches to, 62
  benefits of, 246, 247
  bottom-up, 66, 67, 68, 75, 78, 80
  consultation and, 76
  culture and, 60, 82
  decision-making model, 62, 68
  development of, 5
  discussion in, 65
  dissonance and consonance, 71,
    72
  dynamic nature of, 45

education and, 72, 73, 75, 82
empowerment and, 36
examples of, 75
ideas of, 58
importance of, 143
individual view of, 77, 81
information-sharing in, 65
key ingredients, 81
levels of, 59
Lewin's force field theory of, 64,
    72, 78
liberation and, 88
linear approach to, 63
logic and, 63
management imposed, 58
meaning of, 76
normative-re-educative style, 67,
    72
nurses initiating, 59
nursing and, 58–83
of attitudes, 69, 71, 72, 76
post-coercion model, 74
recognizing need for, 229
resistance to, 43, 65, 77, 82
staff involvement, 80
staff perception of, 76
theories of, 58
three-stage model of, 64
top-down, 66, 67, 68, 70, 76, 82
Chaos theory, 59, 222
Charge nurse:
  primary nurse and, 136, 137
  role of, 135
Choice for patient and nurse, 89
'Chunking', 69
Clinical nurse specialists, 158, 169
Clinical nursing:
  research into, 15, 16
Clinical responsibility, 137
Cognitive dissonance theory, 20,
    70, 77
Cognitive psychology, 212
Collegiality:
  primary nursing and, 133

Common sense, 53
Communication, 213
 role in caring, 234
Communication skill:
 learning, 140
Community care, 79
 nurse practitioners in, 157, 162,
  165, 168
Community nurses, 159
Compassion, 106
Computers in care planning, 196,
  197, 198, 199
Conscientization, 45
Consensus management, 26
Consonance, 71, 72
Consultation:
 by management, 37
 change and, 65, 76
Contract:
 gagging clauses in, 27, 43, 84, 90
Cost containment, 246, 247
Cost cutting, 34, 176
Counselling skills:
 learning, 140
Creativity, 120
Credit Accumulation and Transfer
  Scheme, 172
Criterion validity, 99
Cultural feminism, 28, 29
Cultural myths, 45
Culture:
 attitudes and beliefs in, 61
 change and, 60, 82
 definition of, 60
 environment and, 61
 history and, 61
 homogeneous, 62
 input and output components, 61
 key characteristics, 61
Cumberledge Report, 164

Decision-making, 132, 177
 by doctors, 177
 by nurse practitioners, 177

by nurses, 48
in change, 62, 68
in moral dilemmas, 21
medical, 213
nursing process and, 183
rational, 62
stage model, 211
Delphi technique, 110, 114
Developments, new, 5, 23, 87
Diagnosis:
 medical and nursing, 202
 nursing, *see* Nursing diagnosis
Diploma in Nursing, 15
Discussion in change, 65
Dissonance, 71, 72, 77
Doctors:
 domination by, 10, 11, 42, 84
  education and, 44
 goal of, 51
 nurse practitioners and, 161, 173,
  175, 176
 power of, 46
Domination:
 nature of, 45

Education, 41
 and doctor domination, 44
 change and, 72, 73, 75, 82
 emancipatory teaching, 242
 empowering, 30, 32, 35
 higher, 243
 interactions, 56
 need for, 54
 of nurse practitioners, 155, 162,
  176
 post-registration, 242
 results of, 8
 self-evaluation of, 44
 social control and, 43, 73
 traditional view of, 31
 training and, 7, 23, 30
 ward staff in, 36

Elderly:
  care of, 228–40
    keys to, 236
    statements of belief, 235
Emancipatory teaching, 242
Emergency departments:
  nurse practitioner, 169, 175
Empire-building, 26, 69, 76, 85
Empirics, 21, 22, 31
Empowerment, 87, 106
  as key aspect, 30
  by consensus and collaboration,
    89
  case study of, 229–40
  change and, 36
  collegiality and, 133
  concept of, 25
  control and, 37
  definition of, 25
  feminist perspective, 25–40
  from problem-solving, 74
  in education, 32, 35
  liberated nursing and, 132
  nursing practice and, 41–57
  oppression and, 25
  patient, 27, 121, 177
    nurse practitioners and, 162
    nursing diagnoses and, 204
    primary nursing and, 138–43
  peer-group quality work and, 111
  programmes, 36
  quality and, 114, 119
  reflection and, 50
English Nursing Board Higher
    Award, 160
Environment:
  culture and, 61
Ethics, 21, 105
Experience, 54, 212, 215, 232
Expertise, 55

Female assertion, 12
  male dominance and, 12
Feminism:

central tenet of, 11
consciousness-raising in, 29
cultural, 28, 29
definition, 28
radical, 28
socialist, 28
views within, 29
Financial restraints, 198
Force field theory of change, 64, 72,
    78
Flexibility, 20, 48, 68
Franklin, Benjamin, 59
Freedom:
  loss of, 85
Freire, Paolo, 41, 106, 243, 245

Gender stereotyping, 10, 23, 85
  effect on nursing development,
    14
  effects on profession, 11
General practitioners:
  nurse practitioners and, 167
Gestalt theory, 211, 212, 215
Griffiths Report, 84, 135
Growth:
  empowerment and, 37
  individual, 53
Guevara, Che, 49

Hawthorne effect, 148
Health:
  promotion of, 218
Health budget:
  cost of nurses, 14
Health of the Nation, 96
Health status of patients, 217, 221
Hierarchy:
  obsession with, 61
  primary nursing and, 133
  removal of, 161
  respect for, 60
  vertical, 133
History:
  culture and, 61

Holistic care, 17
Hospitals:
   closure of, 79
   nurse practitioners in, 169, 248
Hugo, Victor, 6
Humanity, 106

Ideas, new, 5, 23, 87
Ideology:
   medical-dominated, 46
Inadequacy:
   feelings of, 35
Information:
   predictability and, 38
Information-sharing, 63
Innovation:
   benefits of, 246, 247
   outcome of, 88
Institute of Advanced Nursing
      Education, 163
Institutional loss, 79
Intuition, 53, 215, 246
   importance of, 216

Job satisfaction, 239
   among nurse practitioners, 158
   definition of, 147
   primary nursing and, 144, 145,
      146, 147, 148
Joint Commission on Accreditation
      of Health Care Organizations,
      193
Junior doctors:
   hours of, 46

Knowledge:
   as power, 28
   attitudes and beliefs in, 60
   base of, 22, 84
   development of, 22, 176
   empirical, 21, 22, 31
   expertise and, 55
   intuitive, 53
   invisible, 52

lack of body of, 9
   nature of, 21
   practice-based, 54, 205
   research and, 14, 87, 244
   then action, 42, 52
Knowledge-based nursing, 20, 21

Language:
   in nursing process, 213
Learned helplessness, 78, 131
   breaking cycle of, 137
Learning:
   experiential, 73
Learning process:
   involvement of students in, 31
Lewin's force field theory of
      change, 64, 72, 78, 217
Liberation, 248
   reflection and, 50
Liberation nursing, 41, 56, 75,
      84–91, 106
   caring and, 86
   change and, 88
   empowerment and, 132
   freedom to nurse and, 85
   nurse practitioners and, 161, 170,
      175
   power and, 86
   primary nursing and, 125, 130,
      151
   providing choice, 89
   results of, 90
Liberation theology, 41
Living activities:
   in care plan, 230
Lovelace, Richard, 84, 90

Male dominance, 10, 11
   care in, 13
   female assertion and, 12
Male nurses, 31
Male values, 30

Management:
  anti-nursing bias, 121
  consensus, 26
  decision-making, 62
  devolvement to wards, 47
  gulf between nurses and, 82
  introduction of, 26
  removing nursing freedom, 85
  size of workforce and, 100
  view on consultation, 37
Managers:
  authority of, 13
  inflicting stress on nurses, 18
  loss of, 12
  power of, 46
Marx, Karl, 41, 73
Medical technology, 46
Medicine:
  nurses subordinate to, 46
Mental health nursing, 77, 191
Messiahs, false, 3, 49, 87, 122
Monitor system, 102, 104, 107
Moral dilemmas, 21
Morale:
  decline in, 27
Myocardial infarction, 218

National Health Service:
  division into Trusts, 27
  future of, 86
  managers, *see under*
    Management; Managers etc.
  number of nurses required, 100
New ideas, 5, 23, 87
New World, New Opportunities, 163
Nightingale, Florence, 8, 33, 42, 90,
    241
Nurse entrepreneur, 47
Nurse practitioners, 125, 155–80
  creativity and, 163
  definitions, 155, 159
  development of, 159
    in USA, 155

  doctors and, 161, 167, 173, 175,
    176
  education for, 155, 162, 176
  fast-track, 170
  flexibility, 163
  impact of, 164
  in A and E departments, 169, 175
  in community care, 157, 162, 165,
    168
  in group practices, 165
  in hospitals, 169, 248
  in primary health care, 174
  in UK, 158
  in-service training, 172
  job description, 170, 171
  job satisfaction among, 158
  liberating nursing practice, 161,
    170, 175
  medical aspects of role, 161
  patient's opinions, 166, 168
  peer review of, 170
  potential of, 174, 178
  recommendation for, 178
  research and, 159, 160, 162
  restrictions on, 157
  role of, 156, 164, 172
  triage and, 173, 175
  value of, 157, 161
Nurse tutors, 44
Nurse–patient relationships, 89, 191
  equalizing, 140
  nature of, 233
  quality of care and, 106
Nurses:
  attitude towards patients, 191
  cost of, 14
  growth and development, 53
  gulf between management and,
    82
  importance to patient, 33
  numbers required, 100
  phases of development, 55
Nursing:
  as female activity, 10, 11

attitudes and beliefs, 18
components of, 56
constraints on, 246
definition of, 232, 233
degree courses in, 15
discipline of, 5
dynamic nature of, 45
future of, 3
intuitive nature of, 21
research and, 15, 16
stereotypes of, 10
subordinate position of, 84
surviving and, 34
Nursing assistants:
  training and, 9
Nursing auxiliaries:
  view of work, 134
Nursing care, *see* Care and caring
Nursing Development Units, 245
Nursing diagnoses, 42, 224
  care planning and, 200
  definition, 201
  financial aspects, 202
  implications of, 216
  nursing models and, 203
  patient empowerment and, 204,
    207
  structure of, 201
Nursing gestalt, 215, 223
Nursing models, 4, 181, 224
  dangers of, 208
  definition of, 232
  development of, 232
  from clinical experience, 232
  nursing diagnosis and, 203
  translating to clinical practice,
    206
  weakness of, 205
Nursing paradox:
  reasons for, 7
Nursing process, 181, 229
  as educational tool, 212
  changing, 210–27
  constraints of, 221

decision-making and, 183
definitions, 181
disempowering patients, 214
from education, 225
identification of problems, 211
individual care and, 190
key words, 182
language of, 213
nurses' understanding of, 184
objectivity of, 214
paperwork involved, 188
quality of care and, 189
  measurement of, 190
research in, 185, 196, 199
task-focused care and, 182, 183
unpopularity of, 186
value of, 210
view of patient, 188
Nursing time:
  use of, 62
Nursing trends:
  compared with sociological
    trends, 135

Obedience, 8
Objectivity, 214
Observation in care, 234
Oppression of nurses, 4, 11, 26, 28,
  42, 132
  empowerment and, 25
Orem's self-care model, 231, 236
Orientation:
  role in caring, 234
Outcome:
  innovation and, 88

Partnership in nursing, 134
Patient:
  choice for, 89
  disempowering, 214
  elderly, *see* Elderly people
  empowerment of, 37, 87, 121, 177
  nurse practitioners and, 162
Patient (*continued*)

nursing diagnoses and, 204, 207
primary nursing and, 138–43
requirements, 139
goals, 69
health status, 217, 221
importance of nurses to, 33
involvement in care, 138, 142
main needs of, 233
nurses' attitude towards, 191
nursing process and, 188
opinions of nurse practitioners,
166, 168
quality of care and, 97, 105, 114
time spent with, 147
Patient problems:
nursing diagnoses and, 203
Patient satisfaction, 116–19
primary nursing and, 146
questionnaires, 118
subjective nature of, 117
Patient-centred care, 48, 117, 121
Patient's Charter, 96
Pay Review Body, 27
Performance indicators, 104
Performance levels, 34
Phaneuf Nursing Audit, 102
Pink, Graham, 113
Politics, 86
women in, 33
*Post-Registration Education and
Practice*, 163, 169, 241
Power, 25
female view of, 26
in politics, 32
knowledge of, 28
male view of, 26
sex differences in view of, 26
traditional view of, 86
use of, 45
see also Empowerment
Powerlessness, 27
Practice:
theory and, 9
Practice nurse, 158

Practice-based knowledge, 54
Practicum, 243
Preconceptions in experience, 54, 55
Pressure sores, 114
Primary nursing, 4, 38, 59, 125–54,
181, 199, 238, 245
accountability and, 131, 136
characteristics of, 129
clinical responsibility and, 137
concepts of, 126
definition of, 126, 144
identification of, 128
implementation, 142, 144
difficulties, 139, 141
importance of, 125
job satisfaction and, 144, 145,
146, 147, 148
liberation of nursing and, 130,
151
nurse's qualification in, 149
organizational model, 127
patient satisfaction with, 146
philosophy of, 150
quality of care and, 148
research into, 127, 142, 145, 148
responsibility in, 136
results of, 143
rituals and, 151, 152
role of ward sister, 136, 137, 141
staff opinions of, 145, 151
staff satisfaction and, 144
stress coping behaviour and, 17
success of, 147
theory and practice, 141
variety of meanings, 130
Problem identification, 211, 227
Procedures:
fondness for, 8
Project 2000, 15, 59, 76, 77, 87, 160,
242, 243
Prophets, 3, 23
Protectionism, 85
Psychology, 211

Quality assurance, 95, 119, *see also*
    Quality of care
Quality of care, 95–124
    aspects of, 122
    care plans and, 187, 197
    definition of, 95, 97
    empowerment and, 114
    external approach to, 96
    financial aspects, 112
    generic measurement, 100
    internal approach to, 96
    involving all staff, 120
    involving compassion, humanity
        and ethics, 106
    measurement of, 142
        audit tools for, 102
        consultations in, 107
        delphi technique, 110, 114
        fallacy of, 103
        in primary and team nursing,
            148, 149
        monitor system, 102, 104, 107
        outcomes, 122
        patient satisfaction, 97, 105,
            114, 116
        peer-group methods, 108, 115
        performance indicators, 104
        Phaneuf Nursing Audit, 102
        quality circles, 109
        Qualpac System, 104
        questionnaires, 110, 118
        reliability of, 97, 98, 99, 103,
            105, 116
        Rush medicus, 102
        Senior Monitor System, 102,
            104, 148
        structure, process and
            outcome, 109
        tools and systems, 102
        validity of, 97, 98, 99, 103, 105,
            116
    ward by ward basis, 106
    numerical representations of, 104
    nurse–patient interaction, 106

    nursing process and, 188, 189
        measurement and, 190
    objective measurement, 100
    primary nursing and, 148, 149
    staff required for, 101
    standard-setting approach, 226
    subjective nature of, 96
Quality circles, 109
Quality of life, 203
Qualpac System, 104
Questionnaires of patient
    satisfaction, 118

Racism in nursing, 33
Rationality:
    change and, 63
Reagan, Ronald, 136
Reflecting in action, 42
Reflection, 56
    as key concept, 49
    liberation and, 50
    role in empowerment, 50
Reflective practice, 66, 87, 162, 185,
    215, 242
    nurse practitioners and, 162
    skills of, 50
Reliability:
    as measurement of care, 97, 98
    definition of, 98
Research, 23, 73, 244
    action, 74, 78
    base for knowledge, 87, 244
    importance of, 14
    lack of, 85
    nurse practitioners and, 159, 160,
        162
    nurses' awareness of, 16
    nursing process and, 185, 188,
        196
    primary nursing and, 127, 142,
        145, 148
Rituals:
    causes of, 22
    defects in, 249

Rituals (*continued*)
  origin of, 6
  primary nursing and, 151, 152
  stress and, 16, 17
  traditional training and, 44
  unnecessary, 18
Role discrepancies, 34
Royal College of Midwives:
  political power of, 86
Royal College of Nursing, 27
  collection of standards, 112
  Dynamic Standard Setting
      System, 96, 108
  political power of, 86
  research by, 15
Rush medicus quality monitoring,
    102

Scientific methods, 21
Self-assertion, 38
Self-awareness, 12
Self-determination, 37
Self-knowledge, 22
Self-perception among nurses, 34
Senior Monitoring System, 102, 104,
    148
Shabbatai Zevi, 3, 5
Shakespeare, William, 60
Sharing, 36
Slater Nursing Performance Scale,
    104
Social control:
  education as, 43, 73
Social sciences:
  nurse training and, 140
  taking over care, 79
Socialist feminism, 28, 29
Sociological trends:
  compared with nursing trends,
      135
Staff:
  calculating requirements of, 101
  involved in change, 80
  reduction in, 27

uncertainty, 66
Staff dissatisfaction:
  primary nursing and, 144
Staffing levels:
  problems of, 105
  reduction in, 200
Staff nurses:
  view of work, 134
Staff training, 115
Standards:
  accountability and, 112
  collection of, 112
  definition of, 108
  ideals of, 34
  peer-group approach to, 108
  setting of, 66, 96, 113
    by professional nurses, 97
    care plans and, 187, 195, 196
    peer-group, 115
    quality of care and, 226
    staff training and, 115
    top-down approach, 111, 114
    validity and reliability, 109
Statistics:
  managers and, 18
Stress, 23
  change and, 74
  defence mechanisms, 16, 23
    attitudes and, 19
    problem-focused or emotion-
        focused, 17
    rituals and, 16, 17
  increase in, 27
  workload and, 18
Student:
  involvement in learning process,
      31
Subordinate groups:
  bringing about subordination, 45,
      46, 47
Supernurse, 158, 159

Team nursing, 136
  hierarchy of power in, 133

Technical rationality, 50, 52
Technical tasks performed by
    nurses, 46
Technology:
    medical, 46
Tennyson, Lord Alfred, 68
Terminal illness, 156
Thatcher, Lady Margaret, 32, 136
Theory and practice, 9, 53
Total quality management, 119
Training:
    apprenticeship model, 8
    attitudes and beliefs in, 18
    cost of, 14
    critical, 242
    education and, 7, 23, 30
    in assertiveness, 13
    linear, 223
    nursing assistants, 9
    origin of, 8
    results of, 7
    social sciences in, 140
    traditional, 44, 185
Trust, 36
Trusts, 27, 47

Unemployment, 27
Uniform:
    assertiveness and, 13
United Kingdom Central Council:
    Code of Professional Conduct, 113

*Community Education and Practice
    Proposals*, 168
nurse practitioners and, 160
political power of, 86
Scope of Professional Practice, 173
United States:
    crisis in health care, 157
    nurse practitioners in, 155

Validity of care measurement, 97,
    98, 99
Values:
    attitudes and, 19
    of nurses, 32, 35, 38
Vanguardism, 49, 53

Ward atmosphere scale, 80
Ward sisters:
    authority of, 43
    primary nurse and, 136, 137
    role of, 133, 135, 141
Ward staff:
    in education, 36
Wards:
    management in, 47
Women:
    in politics, 32, 33
Workload:
    increase in, 27
    stress and, 18

Zevi, Shabbatai, 3, 5